# My Mother's Keeper
## One Family's Journey Through Dementia

S. G. Benson

*Love,*

*S G "Sandy" Benson*

This book is memoir. It reflects the author's present recollections of experiences over time. Some names and characteristics have been changed, some events have been compressed, and some dialogue has been recreated.

*To Barry: Without you I may well not have survived this journey. You were my rock. You walked beside me every step of the way, shouldering the huge burden of helping my parents and helping me help them; consoling me when my efforts fell short. That you did this amidst your own bereavement is beyond amazing. Your kindness and, above all, your patience kept me going when I didn't think I'd make it.*

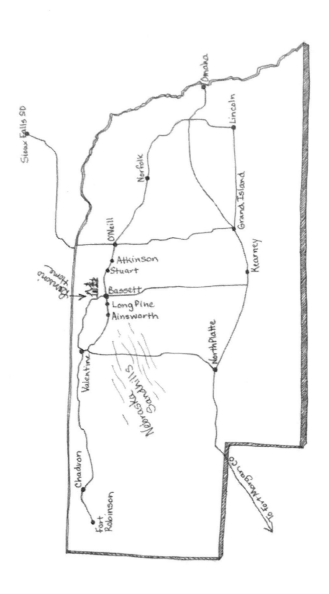

MY MOTHER'S KEEPER

# CONTENTS

# INTRODUCTION

Most people, at some point in their lives, confront issues with aging parents. Whether the problems are medical, financial, logistical, or emotional—or some combination—it's easy to feel overwhelmed and helpless.

When my journey through parental dementia began, I had no idea how much I didn't know. I should have sought information about Alzheimer's disease earlier. At first, I didn't even recognize it as an illness. Once I found myself up to my neck in a nightmare, I had no time for research. I spent every waking moment coping, reacting, and scrambling. I was simply too exhausted to do more than try to put out each fire as it flared.

Later, once the crisis subsided, I found several books, articles, and websites that contained helpful information about dementia, its associated behaviors, and care suggestions for patients. What I didn't find were stories of how families coped with it.

By sharing my experience, I aim to help fill that gap. This book tells my family's story of rapidly-accelerating personality changes, aggression, violence, fear, mistakes, hopelessness, helplessness, and eventual closure. I hope it will help readers who find themselves embarking on a similar journey understand that they are not alone.

S. G. BENSON

# PART ONE

## PROLOGUE
### July 9, 2014—North Central Nebraska

The evening before my sixtieth birthday, my husband, Barry, came home from work and handed me a small package wrapped in tissue paper and topped with a red bow.

"What's this?"

"Open it."

I tore off the wrapping and found a leather-bound journal with a cover featuring a leafy forest. Flipping it open, I saw a binder filled with blank, college-lined paper. A clip fastened a small calendar to a leather pocket containing a calculator. A zippered compartment below held a selection of pens and pencils. An envelope peeked out from a pocket inside the back cover.

I looked up at Barry, who grinned from ear to ear. "Open it."

The card read: "Happy birthday to my favorite forester. I love the stories you bring home from work. Your descriptions of the woods, the wildlife, and the loggers you meet are delightful. Here's a place for you to jot down your adventures, so you can bring me more tales of the great outdoors."

I laughed with delight and gave him a bear hug. "Thank you, Sweetie. I'll take it along with me tomorrow!"

* * *

My journal entries began the very next day. Over the next three years I filled that notebook, but not with what I'd anticipated.

# 1 A DANGEROUS ROAD

**Thursday, July 10, 2014.** This isn't exactly what I'd envisioned for the first entry in my new journal. Today I traveled a familiar prairie highway in my gray, Forest Service work truck at sixty-five miles an hour. As the road dipped into the winding, wooded Long Pine canyon, I slowed to round the first curve.

An elderly man in a battered, blue pickup pulled out from a side road and I slammed the brakes. I sighed and followed him, drumming my fingers on the steering wheel, not daring to cross the double yellow line to pass on that treacherous stretch of road.

I checked my rear-view mirror and saw four more vehicles stacked behind me. Then, a silver sedan. Something about it looked familiar.

Our line of vehicles reached the bottom of the ravine and started up the other side. I glanced in the mirror again and gasped as the silver car pulled out, careened across the centerline, and sped up to pass us all— just as we approached another sharp curve.

"Geez—what an idiot!" I muttered. As the car drew even with me, I looked at the driver. Then my annoyance turned to fear.

*Good God,* I thought. *That's my mother!*

Eighty-five years old, pedal to the metal, she flew by. My ninety-year-old father sat in her passenger seat, pale as a ghost, white knuckles visible as he gripped the panic bar. Mom seemed oblivious to everything as she zipped around the old blue pickup in front of me and swung back into the right lane just as a semi-truck rounded the curve coming toward them. I saw the driver's face, wide-eyed, as he swerved into the shoulder, missing my parents by mere feet.

\* \* \*

*A Love Affair with Driving*

*Mom loved to drive, and for most of her life she'd been very good at it. She got her first license in 1943 at the age of fourteen—and she'd been behind the wheel almost daily for the next seventy years. After retiring, she taught the American Automobile Association's '55-Alive' driver safety class to senior citizens in the town where she lived.*

*Driving meant freedom to her. It allowed her to be on the go, on her own terms, independent of others. My mother possessed a take-charge personality, and self-mobility helped make that possible.*

*As I was growing up, I noticed that when my parents argued, Mom often gave Dad a loud piece of her mind before storming to her car and heading for places unknown. When she returned—sometimes hours later—her demeanor seemed calm. She acted as if nothing had happened. Dad didn't say anything to her about the argument or her departure.*

*When my parents went on long car trips together, they took turns behind the wheel, but my mother usually claimed the first shift to retain tight rein over the route and itinerary. Dad good-naturedly laughed it off, saying that was a battle he didn't want to fight. I didn't even try to get a learner's permit until after I turned seventeen because I knew she'd take me wherever I needed to go. Driving me kept her largely in charge of my comings and goings until I left home.*

* * *

## Cars

*I remember every car Mom had since I was a toddler. She handled her vehicles like a pro, and I always felt safe—even before seat belts. My mother had an instinct to reach out her arm to keep me from flying into the windshield when she hit the brakes.*

*In the days before air conditioning and interstate highways, she'd drive with the windows down and a colorful scarf on her head to keep every hair in place. I remember the scent of the fresh air and the look of pure joy on her face when I accompanied her on the open road.*

*Her early cars were utilitarian, but she had a hankering for a really nice ride— one to match the high life she vigorously pursued. The brand new 1968 black Ford LTD fitted the bill, and I imagine it stretched the limits of her pocketbook as much as it did our little garage. But my parents upgraded to a bigger home in a better neighborhood shortly thereafter, and Mom enjoyed travelling to high-class social events in style.*

*Years later, my mother actually <u>won</u> a BMW in a "Guess the Secret Sound" radio competition. The secret sound was a Ronald Reagan campaign pin sliding into a lapel, and Mom was so proud she figured it out.*

*I remember once, when I came home from college, she allowed me behind the wheel of the BMW—but she never let me start the engine. After I got out of the car, she went in with a polishing cloth and carefully wiped down the steering wheel and dashboard. She didn't want Dad to drive the Beemer, either.*

*About the time my folks retired, frugality replaced extravagance in their automotive choices, and they went through a series of more economical cars. But all of Mom's vehicles were spotless, impeccably detailed, and ding-free.*

# 2 SOMETHING'S AMISS

**Friday, July 11, 2014.** I went to my parents' house after work. Mom's dangerous passing of the line of vehicles on that winding road yesterday worried me, and I wanted to find a non-confrontational way to discuss her actions.

"Did you see me when you passed me on the Long Pine hill yesterday?" I knew I had to be careful because my mother is likely to take offense at any suggestion that her driving isn't up to snuff.

She shook her head.

I took a deep breath. "It scared me when I saw that big truck come around the curve toward you, while you passed so many vehicles."

She glared at me, but softened, probably because she could detect no malice in my facial expression. Then she laughed.

"I've been driving a lot longer than you have, Sandy. I have everything under control. There's no need to worry."

I glanced at Dad, who raised his eyebrows at me but said nothing.

**Monday, July 14, 2014.** I ran into Dad at the post office and he pulled me aside. "I'm worried about your mom," he said. "It scared me, too, the other day when we passed all those vehicles on the highway. She's been taking a lot more risks on the road lately, and her temper has gotten much shorter. She yells at me all the time."

He looked from side to side, shuffling his feet as if fearing being overheard. "I've gotta go," he said. "She's waiting for me."

\* \* \*

*Foundations*

*My mother was born in 1929, at the beginning of the Great Depression, and she came of age as the Second World War wound down. Her parents held prominent social standing in St. Cloud, Minnesota. Her father, a well-known dentist, and her mother, a dental hygienist until they started a family, enjoyed the advantages of high society, including a live-in maid.*

*My mom, Lucy, was the youngest of their three children. She and her sister, Virginia, were young teens when their brother, George, left home to fight in World War II. Mom admired her big brother and when I was small, she sometimes told me stories of his adventures.*

*Tales, like the following one, dominated what Mom related about problems growing up with her sister, with whom she'd shared a bedroom.*

*"You keep away from my side," said Virginia, scowling at her sister, who stood in the doorway.*

*Little Lucy, then maybe six or seven, feared her big sister. The younger girl sniffled, fighting back tears as she eyed the route she'd have to run to reach her own territory. Virginia had built a barrier between their beds, using books and toys to separate her tidy living space from Lucy's cluttered mess.*

*Lucy waited until Virginia looked away, and then scampered as fast as her little legs would carry her across her sister's domain to the safety of her own bed.*

*"Don't be such a cry-baby," Virginia said with a sneer. "And clean up that pigsty!"*

*My mother's feelings of discomfort and unhappiness toward her sister continued for the rest of her life. Years later, Mom told me she did a good job learning to "keep my pigsty clean." I can testify that I never saw anything out of place in my childhood home.*

*Mom told me that when Uncle George came back from the war, he entered dental school and eventually joined his father's practice. She said their parents were dismayed when she announced plans to go into dentistry, too.*

*My grandmother, the picture of poise and gentility, insisted that their youngest daughter learn all the social graces. She and my grandfather sent her to finishing school in Missouri. Lucy hated it, but endured two years there before returning home to attend the University of Minnesota, where she earned a degree in dental hygiene. This breadth of background prepared her well for what she later termed the best of both worlds.*

# 3 HER OWN PARTICULAR WAY

**Saturday, July 19, 2014.** While visiting my parents this afternoon, I paused to admire Mom's taste in decor. Beautiful paintings by well-known western artists hung on the walls, accented by colorful, hand-loomed Navajo rugs. Rare Hopi Kachina dolls sat carefully arranged on well-polished antique tables. Not ostentatious; it just made a subtle statement. The room sparkled from the sunlight streaming in the window. I didn't see a speck of dust anywhere.

I followed the aroma of peach pie and found Mom in the kitchen, peeking into the oven. She smiled. "I invited our priest and a few other people from church over for dinner tomorrow evening. Father Randy loves home-baked pies."

I glanced at a piece of paper on the counter—a menu carefully written in her tidy cursive: Viva la Chicken on wild rice, four-bean salad, dinner rolls, pie with whipped cream. "Mmmm . . . looks yummy," I said. "I know they'll love it."

*She still has a knack for entertaining,* I thought as I headed for home.

**Sunday, July 27, 2014.** Today after church, Father Randy pulled me aside. "Sandy, I'm concerned about your mother," he said.

"Your parents invited Paul, Donna, Chris, and me for supper last Sunday, and something just didn't seem right.

"The food tasted delicious, but throughout the meal your mom continually jumped up and down from her chair—scurrying back and forth to the kitchen, where we could hear her bustling with dishes. I've never seen her do that before.

"Once we finished the main course, Donna got up to help take dishes to the kitchen before I could catch her eye. I remembered that your mother has her own particular way of clearing the table, and I knew she wouldn't welcome the assistance. Sure enough, your mom returned from the kitchen to find Donna holding a stack of dirty plates, and Lucy came unglued. She sternly reprimanded Donna as she took the plates from her hands and marched with them back into the kitchen. Donna looked bewildered and hurt.

We guests all felt pretty uncomfortable during the rest of the meal and—I'm not certain—but I think your dad did, too. Right after dessert, we thanked your parents and left."

"Poor Donna," I said. "I'm so sorry that happened."

Earlier in Mom's life, while she would not have liked having guests help clear the table, she would have had the grace to smile and thank them for the gesture.

\* \* \*

*Mom often said she liked to have me assist her, but doing so proved nearly impossible. A micromanager with a 'Type A' personality, she never seemed satisfied with the efforts of others.*

*I was my mother's best and only kitchen helper throughout my childhood. She taught me to set the table according to her standards, and anything even slightly off earned me a redo. Mom instructed me to place three ice cubes in each water glass. If I put in four, she made me fish one out.*

*Only I could help my mother clear the dinner table because she'd trained me to do it the 'right' way. She said that when people stack soiled plates one on top of the other, the bottoms of them get dirty. Mom scrubbed the plates before placing them in the dishwasher. She hand-washed the most fragile pieces, and when I dried them, she inspected to ensure I didn't leave behind any moisture. I learned to put the clean dishes gently in their correct places, facing the proper direction. After I left the nest, she trained Dad to help her acceptably, but whenever I came to visit, I got my old job back.*

*Mom's pickiness wasn't confined to the kitchen. Often, she'd have a list of jobs for me to do in the yard, garage, or the laundry room. But I waited for her to orchestrate every bit of it because, if I just proceeded with the work on my own, she'd stop me and want it done differently. I distinctly remember performing these chores in increments—completing the first part according to her directions, then pausing and standing stock still until she provided the next set of instructions.*

*My mother worked full time during my school years, so she hired a cleaning lady to come in once a week. When Mom got home from work on those days, she walked through every room to inspect, and she slightly adjusted the position of each item the woman had moved while dusting.*

*I never thought a thing about it until many years later—that's just the way things were done at our house.*

# 4 BALANCING

**Sunday, August 3, 2014:** "I'm sure feeling my age," Dad said when I stopped by my parents' house to reconcile their checkbook this afternoon. I've been doing this accounting for them since January, when Dad asked for my help with it. He told me he just couldn't handle it anymore; by age ninety he'd suffered a series of health scares, and he needed cataract surgery.

Initially, Mom didn't like the idea of my taking over the checkbook duties from Dad, who had always kept track of my parents' finances.

"Why don't you take charge of paying the bills and maintaining the register?" I suggested to her. "I can come by monthly and put everything into the banking program on Dad's computer."

"I guess that would be okay," Mom said. "I don't like using a computer to balance the checkbook, so you can do that part of it."

Mom did a pretty good job with her new task, at first. On the rare occasions I found arithmetic mistakes in the checkbook, I quietly corrected them without saying anything to her. As time passed, though, math errors increased. Once in a while I'd find questionable purchases, but the expenditures were small and I didn't mention them to her.

While I worked on Dad's computer today, my parents sat in chairs nearby. Mom played a game of solitaire, and Dad just watched me and chatted.

"I wear out so easily these days," he said with a sigh, "even though I go to bed early, eat right, and try to exercise. I can barely enjoy a drink before dinner like I used to, because it makes me woozy. I don't like getting old."

Mom looked up and made a face at Dad. "George, stop griping. If anyone should be complaining, it's me. I'm eighty-five. I do all the work around here, and I take excellent care of you."

Yes, Mom has indeed taken good care of my father during his medical issues, and I admire her for that. After Dad suffered a botched bladder-cancer surgery, she chauffeured him to a series of urologist appointments a day's drive from home. She learned to catheterize him and perform other nursing duties that aren't for the faint of heart.

But I'm not so sure about the other ways she 'takes care' of him. I remember last winter, when she insisted that he shovel the driveway immediately after a snowstorm, before my husband, Barry, and I had time to dig ourselves out so we could help them. Overexertion drained Dad to the point he ended up in bed, and she accused him of being a slacker. And this summer she forced him to weed in the yard with her during the hottest part of the day until heat exhaustion nearly claimed him.

\* \* \*

*After college, my mother married, had a child (me), and two years later our little family moved from Minnesota to California. At five, I saw my parents divorce, and Mom and I lived on our own until I turned eleven, when she married George, the man she'd been dating. A wonderful gentleman, he adopted and raised me as his own child. I called him Dad.*

*Our family lived comfortably, with Dad managing a savings and loan and Mom working as a dental hygienist. They were active in their community, volunteering for their church and several charities. They had a vibrant social life. The etiquette my mother learned early served her well. I remember my parents' fashionable dress as they hosted and attended countless elaborate dinner parties.*

*Mom and Dad retired in the mid-1980s and moved to Prescott, Arizona, where they quickly made friends and a mark on their new community with their volunteerism.*

*Dad had a serious bout with bladder cancer in 2003. After a series of operations, my parents and I worried that my mother would soon become a widow. No family members lived near them in Arizona. As an only child, I felt responsible for caring for them. I visited them from Nebraska as often as I could, but between my demanding forestry job and raising a house full of foster children, I found it difficult to get away.*

*On several occasions, I suggested my parents consider moving closer to us, but I never really expected them to do that. Deep inside, I knew the culture shock might prove too much for them. I wrestled with the idea of leaving my job, uprooting my family, and moving to Arizona to care for them—but ultimately, I couldn't make that happen. And so, in 2005, Mom and Dad relocated to Nebraska, which for them was the beginning of the end.*

# 5 OMENS

Our family's situation deteriorated during the rest of that hot Nebraska summer of 2014. Mom became increasingly angry at everything and everybody.

I'd been visiting my parents most weekends for years. I also often dropped by their house after work midweek to see how they were doing and if they needed anything. Although occasionally Mom had a little chore for me, mostly these visits provided a pleasant opportunity to catch up over a cocktail before Mom served supper to Dad.

On one of those occasions, Barry accompanied me. Afterwards, I wrote:

**Wednesday, August 13, 2014:** Mom seemed edgy this evening. She complained at length about how she hates Nebraska and how unkind the people here are to her.

Tired after a long work day, I didn't want to listen to it. I muttered a lame excuse about our needing to get home so I could prepare supper. Looking offended, she started yelling at me. I learned long ago not to yell back, so I just turned and left the house. She followed me out to the driveway.

"Nobody, not even my own family, cares about me," she said, now sobbing.

Barry and my dad trailed us in silence.

Mom threatened me with her fist, and I stepped back to avoid the blow. Without saying anything, I got into our car's passenger seat. I hoped Barry—who had the keys in his pocket—would get into the driver's seat so we could leave. Instead, he stayed in the driveway talking with my parents for a while. Eventually, he calmed Mom down a bit.

\* \* \*

**Summer, 2005**

*Mom and Dad's move from Arizona to Nebraska was rife with omens that none of us recognized at the time. It actually seemed serendipitous, at first. They listed their* house in Arizona, and it sold in just weeks for their full asking price. With his cancer in remission, Dad felt good. My parents worked together on the monumental job of packing up a lifetime of memories.

Our rural Nebraska community offered little in the way of decent housing—my folks couldn't find a rental. But for a reasonable price, they bought a small house just off Bassett's main street, where they planned to live while they built a new home.

In June, I drove to Arizona to transport some of their breakable items. Mom, an amazing packer, had helped me move several times during my younger years. I'd load my car and pronounce it completely full. She'd smile, unpack, rearrange, and shoehorn twice as much into the same space. Now, my mother expertly loaded her most fragile belongings into my vehicle. She told me she didn't want to entrust her china and antiques to a moving company.

The first omen occurred soon after I left my parents' house with Mom's precious cargo. A garbage truck, speeding in the opposite direction, kicked up a big rock that smashed a fist-sized hole in my windshield. I pulled over to assess the situation. The hole sat low on the windshield, well below my normal field of vision. I stuffed a rag into it and continued on my way.

My mother had planned everything carefully. She directed me to store the fragile things at my house in Nebraska. She and Dad intended to follow in a month, when their escrow closed. She said they'd drive both of their Toyotas, loaded with items needed for basic living until the moving van delivered the rest of their possessions. The transport company warned them that, because they were going to a remote and sparsely populated region, their belongings would sit in a warehouse until the movers had a full load to deliver to the area.

Escrow closed on schedule, and in mid-July Mom telephoned to let me know they were on their way. Although I had often made that drive in two and a half days, they—sensibly—planned to make the trip in four.

"We won't be able to take turns at the wheel, since each of us will be driving our own car," she said. "I know your dad can't push too hard. We'll call you the morning of our last day on the road and let you know what time to expect us."

The second omen unfolded the day before I anticipated hearing from my parents about their arrival. A panicked secretary barged into a meeting at my office and handed me a piece of paper with a phone number on it. She told me my mother had called from North Platte, Nebraska, about three hours south of us. "Your mom said there's been an accident and you need to come right away."

*I raced to the phone and made the call. To my relief, the receptionist at the Toyota dealership in North Platte answered the telephone, not someone at a hospital or a police station. She put my mother on the phone.*

*"Your dad hit a deer on the interstate and wrecked his car," Mom said in a shaky voice. She prattled on and on about the damage to the vehicle and how she worried about breakage in the boxes inside, instead of telling me about the condition of my father.*

*I interrupted her, "Is Dad hurt?"*

*"No, the air bag deployed; he's just badly shaken."*

*I called my husband and arranged to swap vehicles so he could use our minivan to transport our foster kids. I drove his little pickup to North Platte in the sweltering July heat.*

*Dad's Toyota was, indeed, badly crunched. The man at the dealership said, "We can order parts, but it will be several weeks before we can complete the repairs."*

*Under my mother's watchful eye and copious instructions, I transferred their boxes from my father's car to the pickup, as Dad observed silently.*

*Mom's car didn't have a square inch of extra space—not even in the passenger seat. We agreed that Dad would ride with me, and my mother would follow us to their new house. That plan fell apart almost immediately.*

*Shortly after we left North Platte, Mom whipped around us and motioned at me as she stopped along the shoulder. I pulled up behind her and walked to her rolled-down window. She asked, "Can't you drive any faster?"*

*"No," I said. "That old pickup won't handle much more than the speed limit."*

*"Well, I'll just meet you at the house," she said, and she went on ahead.*

*The long drive gave Dad and me plenty of time to talk. Still shaken from the accident, the poor man fought back tears, and for nearly an hour he poured out his heart. "Relocating has been really tough," he said. "Your mom has always been high-strung, but she's become increasingly difficult in the weeks leading up to the move. She alternates between hysterical, angry yelling and hopeless crying jags. I'm literally at my wit's end." A few minutes later he fell asleep in my passenger seat.*

# 6 TRYING TO KEEP THINGS MANAGEABLE

**Sunday, August 24, 2014:** My mother's strange behavior is getting worse. Her native sense of decency and propriety seems to be abandoning her. Increasingly, she publicly targets Dad in ways she previously only did in private.

Dad has become stooped-over and unsteady on his feet as he's aged, and he uses a cane now when he leaves the house. In restaurants and at church, Mom loudly scolds him for his poor posture, and it seems like she's constantly pulling back his shoulders, commanding him to stand straight. This morning, during coffee hour after church, I saw her using embarrassing hand gestures while describing to a small audience of parishioners the details of the nursing duties she's been performing since his surgery, such as changing his catheter. Dad stood next to her, red-faced. I quickly changed the subject and guided my parents toward the coffee pot. Mom glared at me.

It appears that my mother is starting to perceive everything as an emergency. Her sense of urgency has increased, and even though my parents don't have a busy schedule, she seems unable to relax. Everything is 'rush, rush, rush.' If Dad fumbles with the key as he unlocks their front door, she swats him on his behind and tells him to hurry. Every time I try to help her with a chore, she leans over me and urges me to move more quickly. When my father sits down to watch the evening news, Mom paces back and forth until she thinks of an activity to busy him.

Dad rarely drives anymore, but he tells me that on the occasions Mom sits in his passenger seat, she harangues him constantly to go faster. It's worse, however, when she's behind the wheel—she relentlessly speeds.

After a couple of nerve-wracking outings with her myself, I've avoided letting my mother drive me anywhere. The last time she rode along with me, I endured a barrage of "hurry ups" and "go fasters."

**Saturday, September 6, 2014:** Dad called me this morning. "Can you please come by the house? Your mom hit me, then stormed into the bedroom and slammed the door. I don't know what to do."

I didn't know what to do either, but I jumped into my car and drove to their home. He met me at the front door and showed me purple bruises on his hands, arms, and legs.

I asked, "Do you want to report this to the sheriff's office?"

"No," he said, "but can we go for a ride and give her some time to cool off?" As we backed out of the driveway, Mom came to the front door and shook her fist at us.

I drove my father around town for a bit.

"I don't know what set her off," he said, "but she attacked me—hitting, kicking, and nearly pushing me down those steep stairs to the basement. I'm afraid of her, and I don't know where to turn."

Eventually, Dad agreed to stop by the sheriff's office, located at the courthouse. "If Deputy Garrett's on duty, it might be okay if we go in and talk to him."

Dad trusts that kind, young deputy, who also serves as a volunteer fireman. For several years he's helped my parents replace their smoke detector batteries.

We found Garrett in his office, and Dad explained what happened. The young man's eyes widened as he listened, and he examined Dad's bruises.

"Do you want to file a written complaint, George?" he asked. "I can't do much without that."

Dad shook his head.

Garrett took photos of the bruises and wrote up a report anyway, just in case my father changed his mind. "Why don't you have your doctor look at your injuries? A physician might be able to suggest some ways to deal with this situation."

Dad asked me to take him home after we left the courthouse. Rather than simply dropping him at the house, I went inside with him to make sure everything was all right. Mom, in the kitchen preparing lunch, strayed from her usual post-outburst demeanor of pretending nothing happened. Instead, she sullenly ignored us.

I decided to stick around for a while.

It was quiet in the kitchen until Mom wheeled around sharply, pointing her finger at Dad. "Don't you EVER go crying to Sandy again," she said through gritted teeth.

"We just went for a ride," I said, deliberately lying. "We wanted to give everything a chance to settle down."

"There's nothing to settle," Mom snapped. "You can leave now." She turned and stomped out of the room.

I looked at Dad with the unspoken question—*should I leave?*

"I think it'll be okay," he whispered.

I wasn't so sure, but he knows her better than I do these days. So, I went home.

**Tuesday, September 9, 2014:** Worried about my father's well-being, I approached Mom and Dad's physician and told him about my mother's increasingly violent tendencies. I asked if there is anything he can do medically to help them.

Dr. Grant looked at me with sympathy. "I wish I could help, but I can't do anything without their permission. You might check with the sheriff's office."

Cripes, now what do we do? Law enforcement said to consult the doctor. The doctor said to consult law enforcement. So basically, everyone says they are sympathetic but they can't help us.

\* \* \*

*In August 2005, Mom and Dad began searching in earnest for real estate once they'd settled into their temporary place in Bassett. They looked long and hard all over north central Nebraska, but could not find a home that offered anything close to the comfort they'd enjoyed in Arizona. The sparsely-populated region contained very few houses at all and almost none for sale. Dad told me, "These homes on the market are old, drafty, and unsuitable for retirement living."*

*In mid-September, Mom and Dad bought a big lot on the hill overlooking Bassett. They settled on a house plan and hired a contractor to construct their new home. They broke ground near the end of October, and my parents stayed happily busy supervising the work all winter, spring, and into the summer. Barry and I helped them move in the following July, and Mom had a ball decorating the house, while Dad oversaw the landscapers.*

*Once the 'busyness' of building, moving, and settling in passed, unhappiness returned. My parents seemed unable to adjust to rural Nebraska life—so very different from what they had known in Arizona. They invited neighbors and community movers-and-shakers to their new home for dinner; very few accepted their invitations, and almost none reciprocated. Mom repeatedly asked me about this. I didn't have any good answers.*

*"I've been here so long, I guess I'm used to it," I said. "This part of Nebraska is just different. People don't entertain at their houses the way they do in Arizona. Around here most folks only invite family members into their homes. School and church activities provide the foundation for the community's social life."*

*That was true, I knew, but I didn't elaborate on the other things I'd learned. They'd find out soon enough that many local residents were unfriendly because they were suspicious of outsiders. Anyone—no matter how nice—whose family hadn't lived there for at least three generations would always be an outsider.*

*Not everyone shunned my parents, though. Congregants from our little church reached out to Mom and Dad and did their best to make them feel included. Several local merchants went out of their way to see that my folks were able to get the products they desired. The grocery store made special orders on their behalf, and the owners of the hardware and appliance store made many kindly deliveries to their house.*

*Two years later, on a summer night in 2008, a tremendous thunderstorm blasted out one of the windows in their sunroom. The rain blew inside, soaking everything. The power went out and Mom, terrified, called 911. The volunteer fire department responded and secured plywood to the gaping hole, as my parents, in their pajamas, watched. That's how they met young Garrett, who became their special friend and protector.*

# 7 SHAKY WHEELS

**Saturday, September 27, 2014:** I got a call from Deputy Garrett this morning.

"Sandy, your mom just had a near-miss on the highway. I saw her stop at the flashing red light by the gas station. Without looking, she pulled out on Highway 20—right in front of a semi. The truck braked hard and nearly T-boned her. She didn't seem to notice; she just kept going. Your dad was in the car with her, and I saw his eyes get pretty wide. I would have pulled her over, if I'd been on duty."

"Geez," I groaned. "Is there anything we can do to keep them—and everyone else—safe?"

"I could send in a report to the Division of Motor Vehicles and ask if they'll contact her," he said.

I urged him to do so.

**Tuesday, October 7, 2014:** Mom phoned me at work today, furious. She said she received a letter from the DMV, notifying her that they are suspending her license until she retests. Since Garrett reassured me that my name would not appear on the report, I knew that her ire, for once, would not be directed at me. I feigned surprise when she told me about the suspension.

"I never had a near-miss with any truck," she said. "Do you know who reported it?"

I sidestepped a direct answer and suggested she contact the DMV with her questions.

"You HAVE to help me," she said in a demanding voice.

"I don't think I can, Mom. But I'll run by the courthouse and pick up a copy of the drivers' handbook for you, so you can study for the test."

**Thursday, October 9, 2014:** I stopped by my parents' house after work to drop off the driver's test booklet. My father met me at the door and took it from me. "I don't think you should come in just now," he said.

This evening I'm wondering how Mom and Dad are doing, but neither of them has called, so I'll stay out of it.

**Tuesday, October 14, 2014:** Today Dad drove Mom to take the driver's exam. He told me later that she fidgeted during the entire forty-five-minute trip to O'Neill. She failed the written test. Once they got home, Dad waited until she went into another room, and then he called me.

"She's absolutely livid," he said. "She screamed at me all the way home. She says she's going to study more, then retake the test. I'm positive I can't drive her there again if she's going to yell at me like that."

**Friday, October 17, 2014:** My mother phoned me at work this morning and politely asked me to drive her to the DMV office on Monday.

"I'm really busy," I told her truthfully. I said it would be hard to get time off during business hours—which might have been a wee exaggeration.

Just before lunch, she called me again, in tears. "Your dad refuses to take me to O'Neill on Monday. Please, please drive me there."

**Monday, October 20, 2014:** I took Mom to O'Neill today, against my better judgment. Because she'd need to take a driving test if she passed the written exam, I drove her Toyota. Mom rode in the passenger seat and Dad sat in the back. Dad hadn't wanted to come along at all, but she'd insisted.

This time she passed the written exam, and the DMV official accompanied her to the Toyota for the driving test. Dad nervously tapped his foot as we waited in the lobby.

Mom marched into the building fifteen minutes later with a big grin on her face. She'd passed, and the official gave her a temporary license, saying she'd receive the reissued one in the mail.

My heart sank. I really wanted to drive them home, but Mom insisted on taking the wheel. I felt relieved to get back to work safely.

\* \* \*

## 1966

*How different things were for my mother's mother. When my grandmother turned seventy, she voluntarily gave up her driver's license. My mom expressed displeasure over her doing so.*

*I was twelve years old and heard Mom scolding Grandma. "Mother, you're too young to stop driving," she said. "Someone will have to taxi you around every time you need to go anywhere. That will put a burden on the family."*

*"No, I won't be a burden," Grandma said. "I can walk to the village if I need something, and I'll take a cab home. Your brother, George, already picks me up for church on Sundays. I really don't need to go out much, and I'm not comfortable driving since my eyesight deteriorated."*

*"Well, I certainly will never give up my license," Mom said, prophetically.*

*Grandma kept her word. She walked to the village weekly and took a taxi home with her groceries. She stayed in good physical and mental shape into her nineties.*

# 8 NOPE, NOT MOVING. EVER.

Mom had several more blow-ups that injured or frightened Dad throughout the rest of autumn and into winter. On a couple of occasions, law enforcement came to their home. Sheriff Joe Harris had issues at the time with his own elderly mother, so perhaps that's why he went above and beyond the call of duty to keep the peace with mine. He and Deputy Garrett were both incredibly patient with her. However, the other deputy, Glenn, wasn't as kind and understanding; when neither Joe nor Garrett was on duty, I made many trips to my parents' house to diffuse tensions.

**Monday, December 1, 2014:** For the moment, we seem to be between emergencies, so this evening when I visited my folks, I gingerly brought up the topic of planning for the future. I reasoned it would be safest to approach the subject in terms of home maintenance.

"This is really a nice house," I began. "Nebraska's harsh winters and hot summers are super hard on it. I know it's getting expensive to maintain, and it's nearly impossible to find anyone to do repairs. Barry and I help but—even with the four of us working at upkeep—things are still slipping through the cracks."

Both of my parents nodded in agreement. So far, so good.

I continued, "Have you two ever given any thought to a retirement community or assisted living facility where someone else is always there to do the heavy lifting? There's a great place in Valentine—that's just forty-five minutes west of here."

I could have heard a pin drop in the icy silence.

* * *

*Mom and Dad had been having the 'whether or not to move to a retirement community' discussion off and on ever since leaving the work force. I remember hearing that conversation for the first time in the late 1980s. Shortly after they moved to Arizona, my parents made a decision not to make such a move, ever. They preferred, they said, to stay in the lovely home they'd built. "We'll just hire help whenever we need it," Mom said.*

*When many of my parents' friends reached their seventies and moved to retirement communities, they raved to my folks about the ease of not having to deal with yard work and outdoor home maintenance. Mom and Dad briefly considered following suit, but again decided against it.*

*A few of those same friends eventually relocated into assisted living facilities. When my parents visited, they had to admit that those places were quite nice. But Mom and Dad said they weren't willing to make such a shift themselves.*

*Not long afterwards, some of those friends transitioned from assisted living into less-pleasant, long-term-care nursing homes, where most of them remained until they died. That seemed to clinch it for my parents. "Nope, we're not doing that, ever," Mom told me.*

# 9 WELL . . . MAYBE . . .

**Monday, January 19, 2015:** Out of the blue, yesterday my parents asked me if I'd take them to Valentine to look at Sunflower Meadows, the assisted living facility I'd mentioned to them last month. My jaw dropped. First thing this morning I picked them up at their house and we headed west. As we made the forty-five-minute drive, Dad told me they'd been discussing my suggestion to consider moving to a retirement community, and they'd decided it wouldn't hurt to at least take a look.

Janet, the facility's administrator, welcomed us warmly and gave us the grand tour. The place seemed clean and well-staffed. It consisted of two sections: assisted living and independent apartments. Janet told us that occupants often started out with an independent apartment and later move into assisted living as their needs increased. She emphasized that Sunflower Meadows was not a nursing home.

"We clean the rooms and change sheets weekly. Residents can receive help with medications, laundry, and even bathing, but when they need actual nursing care, they must move to a place that provides such service," she said.

"Are there any garages?" Mom asked. "We have two cars."

Janet nodded. "There are a few one-car garages on the west end of the building, but they are all currently rented. You'd be second on the waiting list."

She showed us a couple of different-sized apartments, the common areas, laundry, and two well-appointed dining rooms—one of them with a small, private banquet space off to one side, where residents could invite family to gather for special celebrations.

Janet invited us to stay for lunch. Dad seemed impressed with the delicious food, attentive staff, and friendly residents. Mom stayed quiet.

The administrator asked them, "What do you think?"

My mother finally spoke. "I can't imagine how we could fit everything into even the biggest apartment. We'd really have to downsize."

Dad nodded and added, "The cost is really steep."

"Yes," Janet agreed. She shocked me when she said, "We've separated a lot of people from their assets. Most find the trade-off is worth the security, wellness, and peace of mind it offers. Moving to assisted living is not something to enter into lightly."

"Thanks for being honest about that," Dad said.

As we drove home, my parents discussed what they'd seen. They seemed ambivalent, weighing the pros and the cons of what Janet had showed them.

"Do you want to look at other places?" I asked. I mentioned three in nearby towns. "They aren't as nice as Sunflower Meadows, but at least they'll provide some comparisons."

Mom said she had an acquaintance living in a facility in Ainsworth, a town we'd pass through on our way home, so we stopped to visit.

Fairlawn Court looked good on the outside, but the inside appeared a bit run down. The receptionist pointed us toward Mom's friend's apartment. The woman seemed delighted to see us. While everyone chatted, I glanced around the room. Although clean, it appeared tiny, dark, and depressing. *This definitely wouldn't be an option for my parents*, I thought.

**Tuesday, January 20, 2015:** This morning Mom asked if I could get the day off work so we could look at the facilities in the other two towns. After calling both places to confirm that they had openings, I picked up my folks and we headed east.

Sandhills Haven was in Stuart, about a dozen miles from my parents' house. Primarily a nursing home, it also had a small assisted living wing. My parents didn't like it, even though it appeared spotlessly clean and obviously well-run.

"It's pretty sterile," Dad observed.

"It'll be a long time before we're old and sick enough to live in a place like that," Mom said as we continued on our way.

The next place, Cedar View Lodge, was in Atkinson, another twenty minutes' drive east. It struck me as a snapshot of a slower and gentler era. It felt like a large Midwestern home with a comfortable living room and formal dining room. A long breakfast bar looked into a homey kitchen where early risers could enjoy a cup of coffee and chat with the cook while she prepared breakfast. A pleasant porch out back featured comfortable rockers offering a view of a grassy expanse, with a few raised-bed gardens for residents who liked to putter outdoors. Cedar View felt to me just like going to Grandma's house.

The aroma of a baking apple pie wafted from the kitchen, and fresh flowers in vases graced every table in the common areas. The friendly administrator showed us around, pausing first at the dining room.

"There are only a dozen residents here," she said, gesturing to a large walnut dining table. "We dress for dinner and eat family-style."

The rooms were smallish, but bright and clean. Everything sparkled with fresh paint and appeared to be in good repair. We met a few of the residents, who greeted us pleasantly.

Mom and Dad thanked the administrator, and we headed home. They were quiet as we travelled. I wondered what they were thinking, but a little voice inside me warned me not to ask.

\* \* \*

*Little did I know then that the assisted living facilities we'd just visited would soon play an important role in my parents' futures.*

*During that silent drive home, I thought back to the days when my folks had to deal with their own aging parents' living situations. In the mid-1970s Dad's mom, in her late eighties and recently widowed, showed signs of increasing forgetfulness, and her driving became dangerous. Away at college during that time, I never learned the details of how they handled her decline, but she ended up staying in her apartment until shortly before she died. I don't know if she did, but she had the means to hire help to come in daily as her needs increased.*

*My maternal grandmother was the picture of sweetness and refinement. She aged gracefully, even as her health deteriorated throughout the late 1970s and into the 1980s.*

*Uncle George and his wife, Nora, lived just a few minutes from Grandma's house, and they kept a watchful eye on her. Nora, a retired nurse, helped her bathe and monitored her medications. Uncle George made sure the house stayed in good repair, and he hired a woman to come in and clean every Tuesday. My mother, who lived an hour and a half away, visited weekly. She took Grandma to appointments, did her laundry, and brought meals—frozen in individual servings—to last seven days.*

*Although Grandma always treated me wonderfully, Mom complained to me about her. "She's getting hard to be around, and I just can't seem to please her," she said.*

*"There's something I've noticed about old people," my mother told me. "The older they get, the more pronounced their flaws become. Aging brings out the worst in people."*

*How prophetic those words became.*

# 10 THE DECISION

**Wednesday, January 21, 2015:** Mom phoned me early this morning and said they'd decided to move into the first facility we'd visited, Sunflower Meadows, in Valentine. She told me she'd reserved the only remaining two-bedroom suite in the assisted living section, since no apartments were available in the independent living wing. "We're heading there now to get signed up," she said. "We'll tell you all about it when we get back."

I was dumbfounded.

My parents later told me that Janet, the administrator, invited them for lunch before they began the required series of evaluations. I checked the internet and learned that the purpose of such assessments is twofold: to ensure that applicants are physically and functionally able to live at a facility and to establish baseline information that the staff can refer back to over time. Mom and Dad returned by late afternoon, and I stopped by their house after work so they could fill me in on their day's adventures.

My mother said, "They asked me what day of the week it is—and what year. And they had me count by twos and count backwards. That's silly."

"I had to draw a picture of a clock to show what time it is," Dad said. "I agree with your mom; it's pretty crazy."

Nevertheless, they seemed determined to go through with the move. While they were at Sunflower Meadows, they measured the rooms in the apartment, and Mom said she had already started packing.

In a state of disbelief, I thought, *How did they so suddenly flip-flop about relocating?*

"Can I help?" I asked, trying to remember how many vacation days I'd accumulated.

"We won't need anything right now while we're packing," Mom said, "but we will definitely need help moving things."

As I prepared to leave, Dad pulled me aside and asked, "Can we afford this?"

I raised my eyebrows, surprised he'd waited until now to bring up that question. "I'll run the numbers and get back to you," I said.

When I got home, I made some calculations and then called to tell him yes. Barring other expenses, they'd be able to afford assisted living for six years or more, depending on how their investments perform.

"Whew!" he said. "I don't think I'll live another six years, but your mother might."

I'm beginning to feel like we're living in *The Twilight Zone*. The parents I used to know would never have made such a major decision without having all of their financial ducks in a row.

**Thursday, January 22, 2015:** Today I hosted a meeting at my workplace with two forestry supervisors from headquarters. Since usually only my co-worker and I staff the office, I wasn't too surprised when my parents just barged in without knocking.

In the not-too-distant past they would have stopped short upon seeing the visitors, apologized for the interruption, and offered to return later. But times are no longer normal.

"Oh, HELLOOOO," my mother said sweetly, without missing a beat. Dad stood by silently, blushing.

I scrambled to my feet and uncomfortably made introductions. My guests were gracious as they rose and shook hands all around.

"We just dropped in to tell you we're going to Sunflower Meadows," Mom said. "We'll let you know when we get back."

"Okay," I replied as I started herding them from the room.

But my mother wasn't done. "It is *such* a pleasure to meet you," she gushed. As she walked past the visitors, toward the door, she tweaked the cheek of the ranking supervisor.

I cringed but continued escorting my parents to the exit. Returning to the office, I apologized profusely, feeling about an inch tall and wishing I was elsewhere.

\* \* \*

*Later, thinking back to the many times my mother had mortified me over the years, I realized that this latest escapade wasn't at all out of character.*

*One time in 1965, when I was eleven years old, my mother stood on our front step and yelled, "Sandra Jean, you get in here RIGHT NOW!"*

*I immediately detached from my little group of friends and sprinted toward her, hoping to get inside before she further embarrassed me. I didn't make it in time.*

*"Young lady, you KNOW you can't go outside until your chores are done!" She grabbed my arm with one hand and swatted the seat of my pants with the other. I heard my friends titter. For several weeks afterwards, whenever they saw me, they giggled and called me "Young Lady."*

# 11 COUNTDOWN

**Friday, January 23, 2015:** The chaos caused by my parents' sudden decision to move to assisted living is snowballing. I feel stressed and worried, unsure if our family can do everything Mom and Dad need in such an immediate time frame.

Today I took my parents to a bank in Valentine, where we opened a checking account for them. We agreed they will use the new account for local expenses, and I will take charge of their other bank accounts to ensure that bills get paid and their income stream remains uninterrupted.

As if that wasn't enough for one day, after we returned home, my parents listed their house with a Realtor. Please, pinch me! I can barely believe all of this is happening, much less so fast.

**Saturday, January 24, 2015:** Mom and Dad are driving to Valentine several times daily, moving small things. I'm concerned that with all the little stuff they're piling into the apartment, there won't be room for furniture. Today I went to Sunflower Meadows and measured their rooms. I found an online computer program that draws floor plans and furniture to scale, and I gave them the sketch I made to show what would fit in the apartment. I *think* Mom now understands she'll have to make some choices about what to leave behind.

**Sunday, January 25, 2015:** Hoping I'd got it wrong yesterday and that somehow, I'd get a different result today, I went back to the apartment and re-measured more carefully. My parents are going to have to get rid of a LOT of stuff. I asked the administrator, Janet, to recommend a mover. She said the owner of Mike's Market has a large truck and he might be willing to do the job. "We call him Mike the Mover."

**Monday, January 26, 2015:** I called Mike the Mover, and he agreed to haul the furniture for $1,000—but he wants to do it soon, before the approaching snowstorm. We set Thursday as the moving date. I contacted my employer about taking time off. How in the world will we get everything done in three days?

The Realtor showed Mom and Dad's house twice today. One of the viewers made a lowball offer, which my parents rejected.

Things are moving so quickly. My mother continues to pack, turning down my offers of assistance. Because of the time frame, I know I'll have to help her anyway. Mom seems oblivious to the big picture as she focuses solely on packing. Dad appears overwhelmed, although he answers questions when I ask. For the most part, he just keeps his head down and stays out from underfoot.

**Wednesday, January 28, 2015:** I took a day and a half off work to handle some of my parents' pre-move tasks and help pack and transport more boxes—Mom's finally letting me assist with that. Changing contact information for my folks is turning into a headache. It seems like everyone—insurance agents, credit card companies, optometrist, and dentist—needs a copy of the Power of Attorney my parents drew up a couple of years ago, allowing me to act on their behalf. When I accompanied Mom and Dad to their doctor's office for the required physical exams, I had to give the receptionist a copy of the POA before she would switch their billing to me, even though it was Dad who asked her to do it.

At my parents' bank, I changed their statement address to mine, moved funds from savings to checking to handle initial expenses, and set up automatic transfers to start the following month. I sent address notifications for their magazine subscriptions; the post office will forward the rest of their mail to me, so I can pay bills and bring other correspondence to them. I called their accountant about their taxes and arranged for telephone shutoff. I couldn't get through to Medicare—eternal 'hold.' I need to ask Janet at Sunflower Meadows about that.

The neighbors, Allie and Bill, came over to say good-bye. My mother surprised me when she grabbed Allie's hand. "I have something for you."

Mom led Allie to her sewing room and opened the closet door. "You're a talented seamstress. Will you take my sewing machine, material, and all my sewing supplies?"

Allie, teary-eyed, hugged my mother. "Of course." I carried the things across the street to her house.

\* \* \*

*It was much less hectic in 1989 when our family prepared to move my mother's mother out of her home in California. Caring for Grandma after she had a stroke in*

*1988 became too difficult for my aging uncle and aunt, George and Nora, who lived near her. When my parents invited Grandma to live with them in Arizona, Uncle George agreed.*

*My uncle and aunt took care of all the preparations for moving Grandma, which entailed packing the few things she'd need, organizing her financial matters, and adding my mother to the Power of Attorney. They said they'd have plenty of time to settle Grandma's affairs and sell the house once she'd relocated to Arizona.*

*Although we couldn't have known it at the time, the events that followed Grandma's move proved a precursor to my parents' relocation in 2015.*

# 12 THE MOVE

**Thursday, January 29, 2015:** Moving day. What a fiasco! Mom, hyper-stressed and in high-maintenance mode, flitted from room to room, fussing and scolding. Stress-wise, I'm not sure I was in much better shape, but at least I didn't yell at anybody. Thankfully, Barry took the day off work to help, and he proved indispensable—alternating between aiding the movers and calming my mother. Wisely, Dad stayed out of the way.

The moving crew arrived before eight, and it took until early afternoon to get everything into the truck. My mother insisted the men load several items I knew would never fit in the apartment, but she was so distraught that I couldn't talk her out of it.

Mike the Mover touched my arm and whispered, "I'll store whatever won't fit and you can pick it up at my shop later." Mike is more than amazing. He really hit it off with my mother, and she listened to him when none of the rest of us could get through to her.

The crew did a great job loading and unloading the furniture. Nothing got damaged, and most of what they moved actually did fit into the apartment, which became quite crowded. Mike ended up taking several chairs and small tables to storage, but not as much as I'd predicted.

When the movers left, Barry and I stayed at the apartment to help position furniture as best we could, but my mother was so exhausted that she just screamed at us. She seemed convinced that Mike stole her lamps.

"Mom, we only moved a couple of them from your house, and Barry and I brought them in our car," I said—but could tell from the look on her face that she didn't believe me. I assured her I'd bring the others to her tomorrow.

I had trouble getting the checkbook from my mother; she must have forgotten that she'd agreed to let me pay the bills. She finally let me have it, but followed me down the hall to the office when I paid their February rent.

They are sleeping tonight in their apartment for the first time. I'm totally wiped out.

\* \* \*

*Grandma's moving day in 1989 went more smoothly than my parents' move in 2015. The day before, Mom and I drove two vehicles from Arizona to California— Mom in her car to transport her mother and I in my compact pickup to carry a few small pieces of furniture.*

*We overnighted at a motel and arrived at Grandma's house early in the morning. Uncle George had everything packed and ready, and he came to help load. We lifted my grandmother's beloved pair of green chairs, an antique table, and a half-dozen sealed boxes into the bed of my pickup. I covered them with a tarp and tied it down tightly. Uncle George put Grandma's suitcases into the trunk of Mom's car, waved at me, and hugged his mother and sister goodbye.*

*We drove uneventfully across the desert, stopping only for lunch and a couple of bathroom breaks, and arrived at my parents' house in time for supper, which Dad had ready for us.*

# 13 SETTLING IN

More than half of my parents' belongings remained in their house after the moving crew finished their work. Although I believed Mom and Dad now had everything they needed in their new apartment, it soon became evident that my mother did not share my opinion. For the next couple of weeks our days were dominated by packing and transporting things.

**Friday, January 30, 2015:** Mom's in major meltdown mode over lamps. This morning she stormed into my office, asking if I'd called Mike to ask about them. I told her to look in the house first and said I'd meet her there shortly. She'd found some of them by the time I got there, but then she had a huge temper tantrum, holding her hands over her ears and screaming. I was flabbergasted—I'd never seen her behave like that. Neither Dad nor I could approach her, and I had to get Deputy Garrett to help calm her down. *She's totally lost it*, I thought.

Despite Mom's yelling, Dad and I knew we had to get the job done. We packed boxes into their car and mine and took another load to Sunflower Meadows. The apartment is crammed so full that I had to walk sideways to get through the living room.

**Saturday, January 31, 2015:** I met Mom and Dad at their house this morning—they'd brought back a chair that wouldn't fit in the apartment. We filled my car and Mom's with yet MORE boxes and drove back to Valentine. After unloading the vehicles at Sunflower Meadows, I couldn't stay to help unpack. I headed home under a glowering sky, barely beating the incoming storm that Mike the Mover had warned us about.

We've got most of their bedroom stuff out, but Mom wants to come back for kitchen and laundry room items. The apartment doesn't even have a laundry room. Staff will pick up their dirty clothes weekly and return them, clean and folded.

No meltdowns today, thankfully. I got all the lamps moved. What in the world is she going to do with twelve lamps in a three-room apartment?

Whiteout conditions arrived by dusk, with heavy snow blowing sideways. Dad called; they'd left their TV remote at the house. I'm not sure why they need it right away, since their television isn't connected yet. We'll have to wait to get it after the storm quits.

**Sunday, February 1, 2015:** It snowed about eight inches overnight and high winds are making horrible drifts. Church cancelled; everything shut down. Mom called to see how much snow we had and said she wanted to come for another load. I told her it might be Tuesday before we get their driveway plowed out. She's mad . . . again. I'm worried that they might try to drive before the roads are cleared.

I spent the day working via email on more address changes and POA transmittals. I attempted to sign up for electronic access to the new bank account, but couldn't figure it out. I went through their financial files and tried to get better organized. I sense the frustration is just beginning.

**Thursday, February 5, 2015:** The highways opened Monday morning, and Barry and I cleared my parents' driveway. Just as we scooped away the last of the snow from their front walk, the electric garage door opened and Mom's car pulled in. Both Barry and I had to get to work, so we went on our way. I checked on Mom and Dad at noon as they were leaving, car stuffed to the gills. *Where are they putting all that stuff?*

Mom made it clear to me that she's tired of going to the Sunflower Meadows office to make phone calls. I've been trying to get their telephone and internet connected, but there's a waiting list. Today, finally, the company came and got them hooked up. She's already called us three times since supper.

**Friday, February 6, 2015:** I took a day of vacation to start clearing the rest of the stuff out of my parents' house. This is going to be a HUGE job. I'm grateful the folks didn't show up today. They must be up to their eyeballs in unpacking and organizing at the apartment.

I never thought of Mom as a packrat or a hoarder because she always kept everything so tidy and clean. But that house has more storage than any home I've ever seen. There are cabinets everywhere, all completely full. The basement is huge, and each of its three rooms is overflowing. Even upstairs, where I can see they've taken a lot of their belongings to the apartment, there's a ton of stuff left. Besides all the small things, most of their furniture remains. After doing a walk-through, I went to the grocery store and cleaned out their supply of empty boxes.

It's a good thing my mother-in-law's house is just a few blocks away. Barry's mom, Terry, stays there during her summer visits, but she won't be arriving from Florida until May. The house has a couple of empty rooms and a garage where we can store things until we figure out what to do with it all.

**Sunday, February 8, 2015:** Barry and I spent yesterday with my parents. We helped them arrange and rearrange furniture, connect their computers and printers, and set up their TV. We took them to a local café for lunch and they told us about their first week at Sunflower Meadows.

"Early in the morning the nursing aide just walks right into our bedroom to give me my medication," said Dad. "That's a little hard to get used to, but they don't allow us to keep our own medicines in the apartment—even non-prescription meds like my stool softener."

Mom glared at me as I suppressed a chuckle. "It's not funny," she said. "We're not used to having people come in without knocking."

*As if you've never done that*, I thought.

Overall, though, it seems like they are doing okay. For the past several months Mom has complained so much about preparing meals that I'm pretty sure she's relieved she doesn't have to cook anymore, unless she wants to. And Dad actually seems glad to be there.

My mother sent a box of summer clothes back with us, asking me to store them until the weather warms. The apartment still seems awfully crowded, but at least we can walk through it now without knocking into anything.

\* \* \*

*Mom didn't adjust well in 1989, when Grandma moved in with her and Dad. The first week of that experiment was also the last.*

*My grandmother never completely recovered from her stroke, and although she tried to use a walker, she spent most of her waking hours in a wheelchair. Mom scolded her mother when the chair left scratch marks on floors, walls, and furniture. She stewed about having to clean Grandma's bathroom several times daily due to my grandmother's stroke-induced incontinence. Both Mom and Dad complained about getting up multiple times during the night to check on Grandma.*

*My parents tried to solve the problem by giving my grandmother a hand bell to ring when she needed something. "That bell rang constantly," Mom told me later.*

*The following week she placed her mother in a nursing home.*

# 14 A BRIEF PLATEAU

During the remainder of February, March, and into early April, our family's life fell into an uneasy hiatus. Once we got their house emptied, my parents stopped making daily drives to retrieve possessions. I visited them as often as I could.

**Friday, February 13, 2015:** Because I worked in Valentine today, I joined my parents for an early Valentine's Day lunch at Sunflower Meadows. Janet, the administrator, took this photo of us:

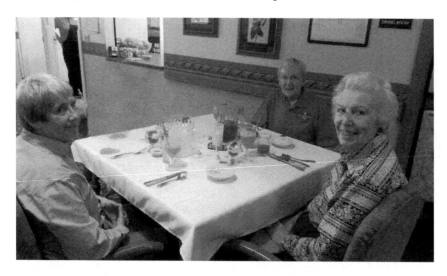

From the picture, one might surmise that things are going great. Not great, I'd say, but as well as could be expected. Mom hasn't lost her ability to smile, and she put on a good act. I walked them back to their apartment after we'd finished eating and said I'd enjoyed lunch.

"The meals here aren't very good," Mom said. "They serve a lot of fried food, and we can't eat that kind of thing—too much cholesterol."

I know for a fact that the facility follows state-mandated dietary standards for the elderly. The meals are planned by a dietician and—from what I've tasted during my visits—the food is prepared by a five-star chef. I also know not to argue with my mother.

**Saturday, February 21, 2015:** Every day after work I've been going to my parents' house to pack and transport boxes and small furniture to my mother-in-law's abode. Barry sweet-talked the FFA kids at the high school into loading and unloading Mom's heavy piano in return for a donation to their organization. Early Tuesday morning they helped us move it to our place. Money well spent. This morning Barry and I took the washer and dryer home to replace our well-worn set. Everything is now out of the house except two vacuum cleaners. Once we're done cleaning, we'll remove those, too. Dad's car can stay in the garage until the property sells.

**Saturday, March 7, 2015:** I'm tired and sad. We are living under a mountain of stuff that needs to be sorted, and much of it must be sold or given away. My mother dislikes Sunflower Meadows, and she's becoming unhappier by the day. But Dad is safer from Mom's outbursts now because there are other people around.

Lady, our eight-year-old golden retriever, died of cancer this week, and I'm having some issues at work.

**Friday, March 20, 2015:** Mom and Dad accepted an offer on their house, and escrow should close in a month. That will be a relief for all of us, but it won't stop their weekly journeys to Bassett to switch vehicles. Barry and I made room in my mother-in-law's garage to store one of their cars.

When I talked to my parents this evening, I learned that Dad's been having fainting spells. I'm glad Sunflower Meadows is just a couple of blocks from the doctor's office and hospital.

Janet told me that Mom takes Dad out in the car every day. Most of their errands are local—medical appointments, shopping, church, or going out for lunch at a restaurant. Mom said today they went to the courthouse and changed their voter registration. I still worry about her reckless driving, but what can I do?

**Wednesday, April 1, 2015:** I stopped by Sunflower Meadows to pay the rent, and Janet asked me to step into her office.

"Your mother isn't adapting to life here as well as we'd hoped," she said. "We've tried getting her involved in our group activities but, frankly, she isn't playing nicely with the others. A couple of days ago, during a game, she started bossing the other ladies around. When they ignored her, she yelled at them and stomped off in a huff."

I didn't mention Janet's comment to Mom. When I entered their apartment, I found her scolding my dad about taking too long to get ready to go out. She immediately turned on me, wagging her finger. "You never should have made us come here," she said. I just bit my tongue.

**Monday, April 20, 2015:** Escrow closed today on my parents' house. Mom and Dad met me at their attorney's office. Virgil Gardner, their lawyer, had the papers waiting for us. My name was also on the deed, so all of us had to sign. My mother appeared to be in sort of a daze, but she nodded politely as we looked over the papers and signed them. Mom seemed to jolt awake when the attorney handed the check to Dad. She snatched it from his hand and dropped it into her purse. Virgil raised his eyebrows and looked at Dad, who stared at his wife but didn't respond.

I said, "Thank you, Virgil."

I turned to my mother. "Let's go to the bank and deposit that money." She nodded and abruptly headed toward the door. Dad hurried to keep up with her.

I collected our copies of the paperwork from the secretary and raced out the door just as Mom's Toyota pulled out of the parking space. I hopped into my car and followed them, breathing a sigh of relief when they stopped in front of the bank.

I followed them inside, took a deposit slip from a stack on the counter, and handed it to my mother. "Do you want to fill this out, or would you rather I do it?"

She gave me a blank stare. "Do what?"

"Get the check out of your purse, and we'll get the deposit slip ready."

"What check?"

"Mom, look in your handbag. You've got the check from selling the house."

Looking puzzled, she unzipped it and rummaged inside. "I don't see a check in here."

Dad's jaw dropped.

"Here, let me look," I said, reaching for her bag. She jerked it away. Two tellers looked up, watching as my mother searched again through her purse.

After what seemed like an eternity, she pulled out the check and waved it at me. "Is this it? Wow, that's a lot of money!"

Dad called me when they got back to Sunflower Meadows. "I didn't breathe again until the teller put that deposit into her drawer," he said.

I can't help but wonder if my mother knows that something is happening to her mind. If she does, is she frightened? Could it be frustration that she is not who she used to be that's causing her increased anger at Dad and me? She hasn't dropped any clues, and I am afraid to ask her about it.

**Wednesday, April 22, 2015:** We're coming up on the *Bargain Buyway* three-day weekend. The annual event is billed as 'The Ultimate Road Trip,' covering 31 towns and 300 miles of garage sales in north central Nebraska. My neighbor, Becky, and I volunteered to spearhead a sale at our church's parish hall, and we spent hours there after work this week, setting up tables, arranging and pricing items. About two thirds of the stuff came from my parents' house. I'm so glad I've had the past month to go through most of their belongings (and Barry's and my junk, too) and separate the 'keep' from the 'get rid of' piles. Becky and a couple of other ladies from church will be running the sale tomorrow, but I'm going to try to get off work a little early to help them at the end of the day. Then, Saturday I'll spend all day there.

*Or so I thought.*

# PART TWO

## 15 EVICTED

**Thursday, April 23, 2015:** Janet, the Sunflower Meadows administrator, called to tell me my mother had kicked my father. Janet took the initial report from Dad and called the police, as she is required to do by law. A young, female officer with the nametag 'L. Wilkins' arrived, interviewed my father, and took photos of his injuries.

I gasped, shocked when Janet said, "Your dad asked to press charges, but Officer Wilkins told us the department couldn't do anything to help him because she determined, after interviewing your mom, that nothing illegal occurred."

The administrator then put her phone on speaker mode. I heard the policewoman talking in a condescending voice to Janet, my dad, and Mardell, the staff nurse. I thought the officer sounded disrespectful. When Janet challenged Wilkins about her tone, the policewoman radioed her supervisor, Lieutenant Barnett. He arrived within five minutes. Although more polite, he backed his officer.

"Even if we could arrest Lucy," the lieutenant said, "the jail would refuse to accept her. They'd have to let her go because of her age and mental condition. We're not allowed to EPC (Emergency Protective Custody) anyone."

The police left the office. Janet kept me on the line while she called the county attorney from her cell phone. I heard their conversation. He seemed sympathetic, but said he has no jurisdiction over the city police department.

After she finished speaking with the official, Janet said to me, "I'm sorry, but we have to evict your mother. As of today, we're giving her fourteen days' notice. I'll try to help you find another place for her. Your father can stay, but it isn't safe for him here now, until she's gone. Please come immediately and pick him up."

The conference call lasted sixty minutes. I spent the next hour on the road to Valentine.

I arrived at Sunflower Meadows about 4:45 p.m. and met Janet and Dad in the administrative office, where I looked at Dad's extensive bruises. My mother sat in the nurses' office where, Mardell told me later, Mom insisted she was justified in kicking Dad because he "yelled and swore" at her. I know that isn't true because Dad is physically incapable of shouting, due to a problem with his larynx. And I have never heard him swear.

Lieutenant Barnett returned to Sunflower Meadows shortly after I arrived and said they could EPC my mother after all—if we took her to the hospital emergency room to be checked by a doctor. At 5:30 p.m. I drove Mom to the ER, and Janet followed us in her car. Janet explained the situation to the receptionist and then left to return to Sunflower Meadows.

A nurse led my mother and me to a small treatment room where we waited over four hours—hungry, because we hadn't eaten anything since lunch. My mother expressed agitation, then sullenness, and finally she demanded that I take her back to the apartment. I told her we had to wait for the doctor. She cried, and when she attempted to stand she swayed back and forth, likely from fear, emotion, and an empty stomach.

About 10 p.m. an obviously exhausted doctor finally arrived and examined Mom. "There isn't anything physically wrong with your mother, so there's nothing we can do," she said. "I'm sorry."

I called Sunflower Meadows. Janet had gone home, but I talked to Mardell. "We have to get your father out of here before we can let your mother back in," she said. "I'll come to the hospital and keep your mom occupied while you pick up your dad. I have his medications packed and labeled for you, and one of the aides put some clothes into a bag for him. He's in the apartment now, waiting for you."

Mardell arrived at the ER at 10:15 p.m. "You've got fifteen minutes to get your dad on the road. I'll settle your mom in for the night. Call me in the morning."

I found my father sitting at the kitchen table in the apartment, crying. I hugged him, grabbed his overnight bag, and led him to the door. I picked up his medications at the front desk as we left. We didn't talk much during the trip to my home—I think we were both in a daze. We got to the house about midnight. Barry had waited up for us, and he helped me get Dad settled into the guest room.

Tonight, my father and I are utterly exhausted.

**Friday, April 24, 2015:** Dad woke by six, and I gave him his medications before breakfast. The phone rang at a quarter to seven. Mom's voice sounded tense, yet distant, as she asked to speak to her husband. I looked at my father, and he shook his head. "He's in the bathroom," I lied. "I'll give him the message."

Barry headed off to work, leaving Dad and me alone for the day. This is alien territory for me, and I must figure out a plan of action. I don't even know where to start.

Today, Arbor Day, is a state holiday in Nebraska, but it's always a work day for me, so I had to use some vacation leave. I knew it would be tough to get much done, though, because businesses and state government offices would be closed. At 8 a.m. I started making phone calls, as Dad watched and listened.

First, I called my workplace and asked my co-worker to cover for me. "Please disregard any phone calls my mother makes to our office. If you do pick up and she asks questions about anything, just offer to take a message."

Then, I reached out to my parents' attorney. I described the situation and asked if he could guide us. He said his legal work is mostly limited to real estate closings and county business. He recommended we contact a lawyer who has a broader area of expertise.

Next, I called Warren Arganbright, an attorney in Valentine. I left a message on his answering machine, briefly explaining the situation and asking about our options. To my surprise, he returned my call.

"We'll need to get an emergency protection order for your dad, and then you should look into getting guardianship of your mother so you can move her into an Alzheimer's' care facility. There isn't much we can do today because of the holiday."

We set an appointment for Dad and me at Warren's office on Monday. It looks like we'll be on our own for the long weekend.

I phoned Mardell at Sunflower Meadows as I'd promised. She said Mom got up early but so far had stayed in the apartment, waiting for Dad to return her call. "Janet's been contacting other facilities in the area, trying to find one with an opening that is willing to accept your mother."

As soon as Mardell and I finished, my mother called and demanded to speak with Dad. Again, he shook his head.

"Mom," I said, "he doesn't want to talk to you right now."

She snorted and hung up.

After lunch I took my father to the church, where we helped with the rummage sale. It kept us distracted from the emergency and Dad said it pleased him to see that some of their things had already sold.

When we returned home we found a note from Mom on the front door. "Where were you today? I came twice, but couldn't find you."

I looked at my father. "I'm sure glad we locked the house when we left!"

Dad nodded, apparently making some mental calculations. "Two trips here from Valentine tells me she must have been on the road for at least four hours today."

We found a dozen messages from Mom on our answering machine, ranging from angry tirades to pleas for my father to talk to her. He refused. During the evening she called several more times, but we let it go to voice mail. We unplugged the phone when we went to bed.

# 16 COPS AND ROBBERS

**Sunday, April 26, 2015:** Dad and I spent the entire weekend hiding from my mother, who was actively stalking him. Yesterday, Mom began calling at sunrise, and she didn't let up. I picked up the phone a few times, but found it impossible to communicate through her screaming and tears. Once I stopped answering the phone, I knew it would be just a matter of time before she got into her car and headed our way. My father and I went to the church and helped with the sale.

After lunch, I took Dad to my mother-in-law's house for a nap, telling him to keep the door locked and not answer if anyone knocked. I hid my car behind a neighbor's fence and walked the block to the parish hall to take another shift.

Not ten minutes later, Mom appeared in the church's doorway, looking around until she spotted me. She strode with purpose to the cashier's table where I sat.

"Where's your father?"

"He isn't here."

"I can see that. Is he with Barry?"

I shrugged and handed her a bottle of water from my cooler. "You must be tired from that long drive. Do you want to look around? You have a lot of things here, and some of them have sold already."

"What are you going to do with the money?"

"Ten percent goes to the church. We'll put the rest into your checking account."

She looked relieved, took a sip of water, and began walking about, examining the merchandise. Halfway down the middle aisle she stopped and picked up an ordinary-looking wine decanter. "That's mine! You can't sell this." She tucked it into her large handbag and continued on, stopping here and there to add items to her collection.

When she finished, she returned to the front table. "I'm going to look for your father. If he comes back, tell him to stay here until I return." She left, purse bulging with her reclaimed possessions.

Guessing she would go to my house, I calculated we'd have forty minutes before she returned. I stayed another twenty minutes and then went to my mother-in-law's house to get Dad. I unlocked the door and found him just waking up from his nap.

"Mom's in town, looking for you."

"I don't want her to find me. Can we go see Garrett at the sheriff's office?"

I backed my car out of its hiding place and my father climbed in. We drove the two blocks to the courthouse, and I parked in the shade of the building, leaving the engine running and the air conditioner on because the April sunshine felt hot. "You stay here and keep the doors locked," I said. "I'll see if Garrett is working today."

Dad flashed an odd smile. "This is just like playing 'Cops and Robbers,' but it's no game."

I found the dispatcher alone in the office. She said, "Garrett's off-duty, but I'll call Glenn if you need a deputy."

I thought for a moment. "No thanks. Glenn has little sympathy for our family's situation."

Back in the parking lot, Dad pushed the 'unlock' button and I got into the car—just as Mom's Toyota pulled into the driveway. Quickly, I relocked the doors.

She stopped next to us and got out, glaring at her husband. "What do you think you're doing?"

He didn't answer, which appeared to further enrage her.

There were no other cars in the lot, and on that side of the building there are no windows that might have allowed the dispatcher to observe us and call for help. I slipped the transmission into reverse and began easing out of the parking spot. Mom, screaming, pounded her fist on my car, but I continued backing until I could turn toward the exit.

I held my breath as we moved slowly away from her—then sped up, once I could be certain I wouldn't accidentally run into her. We turned the corner before she could get back into her car to chase us. I headed out of town in the opposite direction from the way home, pulled off on a side street, and hid.

Today wasn't much better than yesterday. From my calculations, Mom spent at least six hours each day driving between Valentine and Bassett, and—when she wasn't on the road—she was on the phone screaming into the answering machine. Tonight, Dad and I are pooped. I'm really glad we've got that appointment with the attorney tomorrow.

# 17 PROTECTION ORDER

**Monday, April 27, 2015:** My father and I spent the day scrambling to protect him from my mother's stalking and violent behavior. Over the weekend, Mom threatened to clean out their savings. I took Dad to the bank early and, as the primary holder, he removed her name from my parents' accounts.

We then drove to Valentine and met with attorney Arganbright. He'd prepared a protection order for my father and an emergency request asking the court to grant me temporary custody of my mother until they can hold an official guardianship hearing. The judge approved both. The lawyer delivered the papers to the police department secretary, who said an officer would serve them to my mom tomorrow. I called Sunflower Meadows to let Janet know they'll be coming.

She thanked me and said that Cedar View Lodge, in Atkinson, agreed to take my mother—if she passes both a physical exam and their social worker's assessment. I made a doctor appointment for Mom. If that goes well, she could move by Thursday.

Meanwhile, my mother drove back and forth several times between Valentine and our house today, presumably trying to find us, but we eluded her. I checked my work email before bedtime. My co-worker said she saved a message from my mom on the answering machine. I hope we don't have to use these messages in court, but I'm keeping them in case we do.

**Tuesday, April 28, 2015:** This horror movie just keeps getting worse. Barry took the day off to stay with Dad. I left for my office just before sunrise, needing to catch up on work. As I headed toward town, a silver Toyota passed me, going the other direction. It looked like Mom's, but I couldn't see it clearly in the dawn haze. *She wouldn't leave Sunflower Meadows until it gets light,* I thought. I chalked it up to my imagination and went on to work.

Barry called as I walked into my office. He said that shortly after I left, my mother pulled into the driveway, stomped loudly up the stairs to the porch, and pounded on the front door. "Fortunately, we had everything locked. George and I hid. She just left a few minutes ago, so you might watch for her."

I kept my office door locked until I left at 8:15 for a meeting in Valentine. I alerted my boss that I'd be taking vacation time after the meeting and likely for the rest of the week.

On my way out of town, I stopped for gas. The guy who runs the station said Mom had been there at daybreak, filling her tank. He asked, "Is Lucy okay?"

My mother beat me to Valentine. I stopped at Sunflower Meadows to pick up Dad's prescription refills, and through the glass front doors I saw Mom pacing the lobby. I knocked on Janet's office window and asked her to send someone out with the meds.

After my meeting, I took my mother to her doctor's office in Bassett. She cried, yelled, ranted, and raved the whole way. Once, she threatened to get out of the moving car, but she didn't undo her seat belt, so I kept driving. I counted seven suicide threats on the way to Bassett and three on the way back to Valentine. Dr. Grant gave her a new prescription and told her if she didn't take it she wouldn't have a place to move to. They faxed the Rx to both Sunflower Meadows and the Atkinson facility, but based on what I learned next, my guess is she didn't take it.

After dropping Mom at Sunflower Meadows, I checked with the police department to see if Dad's protection order had been served. The dispatcher said the officers were unable to find my mother, although they'd tried several times. I left Valentine about 5:30 p.m. and headed home.

Mom beat me back to our house, but she'd left by the time I got there. Barry said she'd been sneaky and almost caught him and Dad. "She parked way up the driveway and walked to the house so we wouldn't see her car. We ducked into a dark hallway before she saw us. She walked all around the house, looking in the windows and trying every door. She left a half carafe of red wine on the porch. We dumped it down the sink, not knowing what she might have put in it."

This means my mother spent six hours on the road today, including the two hours in the car with me. Three trips to Bassett—6 a.m., 2 p.m., and 6 p.m., and she missed both breakfast and supper at Sunflower Meadows. I'm wondering if she is eating.

**Wednesday, April 29, 2015:** I'm worried about Dad. Last night he got up to use the bathroom and bumped his shin on a table. Bleeding, he came to our room and asked for a Band-Aid. I keep the kitchen light on at night to help him see if he leaves his bedroom, but our house really isn't set up for the elderly, and I'm not confident in my ability to provide elder care.

First thing this morning, Janet called from Sunflower Meadows. "Cedar View Lodge can do your mother's assessment today. I know you've got your hands full with your dad, and you likely won't be able to take her to Atkinson. Our cook, Ron, offered to use his day off and drive her in his own vehicle to the appointment. I'll call you afterwards to let you know what happened." When we hung up, I told my father what she'd said.

Dad smiled. "Ron's a good man. He's taken a liking to both Lucy and me, but I never expected him to do something like this. I need to thank him."

Father Randy phoned a few minutes later to see how things were going and offered to help. He said he called my mother yesterday evening, and she didn't sound good.

Needing a little pastoral consolation myself, I said, "Mom says you never call her, but I know you do. Yesterday, Barry and I spent fourteen hours trying to help her get approved by Cedar View Lodge, and today we both took another day off work to keep Dad out of harm's way. All of us are worn out. This nightmare has to end soon, or we'll go crazy. I'll find out today if we can move Mom tomorrow. I'll let you know if we need your help."

Janet called back around noon and said Mom passed the social worker's assessment. "I had to assure her that Lucy's only a danger to George and not to anyone else. She hasn't started packing yet, and we want her out tomorrow. Can you help get her going on this?"

Mom answered her phone on the first ring. I asked if I could help her pack. She screamed something unintelligible and slammed down the receiver.

I called Mike the Mover and he agreed to move her tomorrow.

"Mom's angry and she won't let me help her pack," I told him.

"I'll give her a hand with that tonight," he said.

Janet checked in with me at 2:45 p.m. "The police served the papers to your mother. She is blaming you, so you probably shouldn't attempt to see or phone her. We'll try to calm her down."

It was almost 8:30 p.m. when I finally heard from Mover Mike. "We got your mom all packed, but she's going to need a smaller bed—didn't you say you have one at your house? The only way she'll agree to leave is if she can drive her car tomorrow. The plan is for Lucy to follow me to Atkinson, and once we get unloaded, I'll see if I can convince her to let my helper take her vehicle back to Bassett, since she will think it needs repairs. I disconnected the battery tonight so she can't go anywhere."

He chuckled. "I'll get it going for her in the morning and tell her not to turn off the engine because it may not start again."

Mike echoed Janet's warning when he advised me not to show up at Sunflower Meadows tomorrow to help; he said to just meet him in Bassett with the bed.

*Good God, this whole situation is awful.*

# 18 CAR TROUBLE

**Thursday, April 30, 2015:** Nurse Mardell phoned early and said, "Your mother came to the office in a tizzy when her car wouldn't start. But Mike the Mover got it running and drove it around back. It looks like he and your mom are putting things in both his van and her car."

As he led Mom out of Valentine, Mike called to tell me they were on their way to meet me to get the bed.

Barry helped me load a twin bed into his truck. He stayed home with Dad while I drove the pickup to Bassett, where the mover and my mother waited. She ignored me as Mike and I transferred the bed to his van. I followed them to Cedar View Lodge in Atkinson.

After we unloaded Mom's belongings, Mike tried to persuade my mother to let his helper take her car back to the mechanic in Bassett. She refused. After she went inside the building, Mike removed a fuse from her Toyota and handed it to me. I put it in my pocket, and on my way home I gave it and the spare key to friends from our church. They agreed to 'steal' the car tomorrow (perfectly legal, now that I have custody of Mom). I told the Cedar View Lodge staff what I'd done and why.

When I got home, I dialed Mardell at Sunflower Meadows. "We got Mom moved in; we're leaving her to unpack. Dad and I will see you in the morning. We'll take inventory and see what she left him. My mother won't be visiting you any time soon. Strangely, her car has stopped working."

"Yes, I may have heard a rumor she was having car troubles—hopefully she doesn't call the local garage to have it fixed. I'm excited to have your dad back with us!"

**Friday, May 1, 2015:** Julie, the Cedar View Lodge administrator, phoned early. "Your mother couldn't start her car, and she's begun calling repair shops. We tipped off the local mechanics to make sure they won't help right away."

A few minutes later, Mom called me, and I told her I'd get it fixed. Tonight, after dark, my friends went to her car, put the fuse in, started it, and drove it to their garage.

Dad is settled in once again at Sunflower Meadows. The staff greeted him warmly when I dropped him off, and he seemed genuinely happy to be there again. I told him I'd visit soon.

My mother is already wearing out her welcome at Cedar View Lodge. The employees tell me she constantly asks other residents to borrow their phones. I'm not sure what to do. I called Attorney Arganbright and said I'm worried that if she gets thrown out of there, I have nowhere to put her. He suggested I check with the behavioral health clinic in Kearney. It's after hours now, but I'll call them Monday.

**Saturday, May 2, 2015:** Mom called me this morning. "My car's gone."

"Don't worry. I had it towed to the repair shop." Lying came easier this time, but it still left me with a twinge of guilt.

Barry gave me a ride to our friends' house. I fired up my mother's Toyota and drove it to Bassett, where I stashed it in my mother-in-law's garage.

I keep our landline unplugged most of the time because of Mom's constant pestering. I told her to stop using other people's telephones and that I'd give her back her flip phone—if she'd promise not to call me after eight in the evening. Because it's so hard to talk to her, I left her a letter explaining why she had to move and expressing my hope that she will adjust to her new surroundings. I feel like a monster. But what can I do?

# 19 MOTHERS' DAY

**Tuesday, May 5, 2015:** Barry drove to the Grand Island airport today to pick up his mother, Terry. She'll be at her house in Bassett for the summer. Last night we dusted and vacuumed it and turned on the refrigerator, so everything is ready for her. We know she'll be surprised to see my mother's car in her garage. Barry said that during the trip home from the airport he brought his mom up to speed on what's been happening with my parents. I really hope this summer won't be difficult for her because of it.

**Thursday, May 7, 2015:** I've been thinking that my mother may be getting settled in to her new surroundings. I plugged our telephone back in yesterday, and she hasn't called—is that a good sign?

This afternoon, Julie, the Cedar View Lodge administrator, said, "Your mom went outside for a walk today. When she returned, she reported that she got lost, and a gentleman gave her a ride back to our facility. She told me that when she gets more familiar with this area she won't get disoriented again. But I'm leaving it up to you to decide if it is safe for her to go out walking alone."

"I'm surprised she got confused—she knows her way around Atkinson. When I see her Sunday, I'll try to get a handle on her condition and get back to you on Monday. She may be deteriorating faster than I think. For now, walks are okay."

"That's fine. I'll have you sign a form stating that you're aware of the risks. Otherwise, we can change the resident service plan to state she isn't authorized to leave the building unsupervised."

**Sunday, May 10, 2015:** Mothers' Day. Father Randy brought Mom to church, and afterwards Barry and I took our mothers to lunch. Mom spoke rudely to Terry, and she bad-mouthed Dad. When I took my mother back to Cedar View Lodge, I said I'd see her next Saturday—although I'm beginning to think it might be better for her if I did not visit at all. She's still pretty angry with me.

I stopped at Terry's house on my way home to apologize for the way my mother treated her. My mother-in-law is the kindest, most compassionate person I've ever known. She reminded me that my mom isn't the person she used to be and that we all must try to be understanding and patient.

During our visit, Terry said, "This will likely be my last trip to Nebraska."

Thinking she said this because she found it difficult to change planes in the busy Dallas/Fort Worth airport, I said, "Next year let's route you through Sioux Falls—that's non-stop."

She said no, it's not that, but didn't go into more detail. I mentioned it to Barry when I got home, and he said he'd talk to her.

# 20 EVICTED, AGAIN

**Monday, May 11, 2015:** Last night Dad told me that Mom has been calling him repeatedly and threatening him.

This morning I spoke with Julie. "My mother violated my father's protection order by harassing him. Next weekend, I will take away Mom's mobile phone and tell her she must not borrow anyone else's."

Warren Arganbright, the attorney, inquired if my father wants to cancel Friday's protection order hearing, now that my mother doesn't have her car. When I asked Dad about it, he said, "No, please don't do that. I'm afraid she'll find a ride back to Valentine, and I just can't handle her hitting me anymore. Did you tell Warren that she's been calling and screaming at me?"

"Yes, Dad, I did. I'll pick you up at nine-thirty Friday morning to take you to the courthouse."

"Is Lucy going to be at the hearing?"

"I don't think so, but I'll check with Warren."

When I contacted the law office, Warren described how protection orders work. "If your mother wants a hearing, she must request it by signing the form she got when the police served her the papers and then filing it with the court. If she does NOT sign and file, the court can ask for a 'show cause' hearing, whereby your mother has to explain why the order should not remain in effect for one year. If she does not appear, the protection order becomes final. Whether or not you bring her to the hearing is up to you. If she does appear, she has to testify. But I still want your dad there, just in case."

Mom has not signed and filed papers regarding the hearing. I am certain that she doesn't understand this process. Even after the explanation, I barely do. I've decided not to bring her to court.

**Tuesday, May 12, 2015:** Julie called me this morning. "Last night your mother assaulted another resident and took his phone. When an employee intervened, Lucy threatened to slit her wrists. She denies it happened, but our staff documented the incident. We did not report it to the police, but we must evict her. She has thirty days to get out. I asked Dr. Grant for a stronger prescription to calm her aggression."

The receptionist at Dr. Grant's office confirmed that they faxed a new prescription to the pharmacy. The drug is called "Abilify" and the co-pay is steep. It's not on the list of medications covered by Mom's insurance.

Where can I put her? I've contacted all of the other assisted living facilities in this part of the state. None of them will take a demented person with violent behavior.

I sought Warren's advice. He said, "Instead of looking for another assisted living facility, how about focusing on finding a nursing home with an Alzheimer's unit?" He suggested one in North Platte, but when I checked with them, they informed me they can't handle people with behavioral problems. They recommended another place, in Fort Morgan, Colorado. I tried them, but they have no openings. I called facilities with Alzheimer's units in Stuart, Gothenburg, and Fullerton, Nebraska, but they were all full.

Finally, I got through to the behavioral health clinic in Kearney that Warren mentioned last week. They only take admissions through psychiatrist referrals. They recommended a hospital in Lincoln, but, when I contacted them, they told me the same thing. I looked through the yellow pages for psychiatrists. There aren't any nearby, and the two I contacted in Grand Island have no openings this month. As a last resort, I checked with the Atkinson Police Department, hoping they might be able to recommend someone to assist me. The officer said that since Cedar View Lodge didn't request their assistance, there was no police report of the incident—which means they can't help, either.

I'm running out of options. I'm afraid they will just put her out on the street if I don't come and get her. I can pick up her stuff, but I can't handle her behavior any better than they can. Is there anything anyone can do?

**Wednesday, May 13, 2015:** Julie told me that Mom took another walk yesterday and got lost again. "I've been networking to help you find a place for your mother. I just learned the Four Seasons Nursing Home in O'Neill has a new opening in their Alzheimer's unit."

I immediately phoned the nursing home and talked to a caseworker, Diane. She agreed to travel to Atkinson in the morning and do an assessment on Mom. I'll go look at the facility tomorrow. If they accept her, I'll move her as soon as possible. If not, we are back to square one.

I'm out of vacation time and have asked my employer about taking leave without pay. They are helping me look into emergency family leave instead—I'm grateful.

**Thursday, May 14, 2015:** This morning, Julie said, "Dr. Grant referred Lucy to a geriatric psychiatrist in Omaha, but he doesn't have an opening until October. I told them it's an emergency, and they arranged to do a 'tele-health' appointment May 28th at the outpatient clinic in O'Neill. You'll have to be there with her so the doctor can ask you questions. I'm mailing you some paperwork you'll need to fill out and return to me right away."

When I stopped by Dr. Grant's office with some questions about Mom's medication, I felt fortunate to catch him in person instead of having to talk to a nurse.

"Mom has always been on top of everything. How could this dementia have happened to her so suddenly?"

"It's probably been coming on gradually—it only seems sudden," he said. "It's likely your mother did an expert job covering up her diminishing capabilities—especially considering she doesn't understand what is happening. She fooled all of us, until one day she just couldn't cover any longer—and then it all came out at once. I'm sorry that you and George have to deal with this. It's hard on both of you."

I drove to O'Neill and checked out the Four Seasons Nursing Home. The place isn't great; it looks pretty clean, but the halls smell of excrement and disinfectant. At this point we can't be picky. I stopped to see Mom when I passed through Atkinson on my way home. She told me that she likes Cedar View Lodge now and that Julie is letting her stay there. Of course, I checked with Julie, and no, she has thirty days to get out.

The phone rang as I got home. I cringed when I heard Mom's voice.

"I walked over to Father Randy's house. He isn't home, but he left the door unlocked. I don't think he'll mind that I'm using his phone."

She went on and on about the same old stuff: how she wanted to see George—but all of this was his fault—and how lonely she felt. With a twinge of guilt, I finally just hung up.

I feel sorry for her, but talking to her doesn't seem to help.

**Friday, May 15, 2015:** I drove to Valentine and took my father to court. The judge extended the protection order for a year. Dad did a good job testifying, but it obviously exhausted him.

Afterwards, I bought him lunch, and we went shopping for a few necessities. Dad asked me to push him in the store-provided wheelchair. He is really getting feeble.

When I got home, I called Diane at the Four Seasons Nursing Home. She said she did the assessment on Mom, and the facility will take her. I am relieved; the trick will be getting her to go!

# 21 ANOTHER MOVE

**Saturday, May 16, 2015:** My neighbor, Becky, accompanied me to visit my mother today, because I knew it wouldn't go well if I went alone. It didn't go well, anyway. We brought Mom some boxes so she can start packing, but she doesn't understand that she has to move again, and she's convinced none of this is her fault. I refused to have that discussion.

We took my mother downtown to buy a few things she wanted, but that proved crazy and difficult. She even got mad at Becky, so I considered it a wasted trip. I told Mom to get packed, and we'll be back on Tuesday to move her.

I'm worried about money. So far the legal bills are over $1,200. The invoice from the pharmacy for the co-pay on her new prescription is another $400. I looked at the literature from the Four Seasons Nursing Home, and the room will cost over $6,500 a month, more than twice the rent at Cedar View Lodge. Plus, we're still paying $3,500 monthly on Dad's apartment at Sunflower Meadows. It won't take long to go through their savings. Damn.

**Sunday, May 17, 2015:** I drove to Valentine this morning and took Dad to church, then out shopping for a few items he needed. After lunch I fixed some problems on his computer. We had a good day, and it made me happy to see him smiling.

When I returned home, my husband told me that he took his mom to our church in Bassett. Father Randy picked up my mother and brought her to the service, where he seated her next to Barry.

"Lucy ignored my mom, tried to butter me up, and she announced to the congregation that recently a police officer stopped her to compliment her on her excellent driving skills." He sighed. "She also told me to tell you that if you don't return her car, she will ask the sheriff to make you give it back. She spent a lot of time badmouthing you."

I'm glad I missed that.

Barry said he's worried about his mother. "When I suggested making easier flight arrangements for next year's visit, Mom told me she hit her head on a shelf at home in Florida and has been having headaches ever since. I promised I'd make an appointment for her at the clinic this week."

**Monday, May 18, 2015:** I told my boss I won't be at work tomorrow because we're going to *try* to get my mother moved from Cedar View Lodge in Atkinson to the Alzheimer's unit at the Four Seasons Nursing Home in O'Neill. Right now, Mom's refusing to pack—but if I can somehow get her there, I can return to the apartment and box her stuff myself. I'm hoping to recruit Deputy Garrett, who told me he's off-duty that day, to help persuade her.

After lunch, Julie reported that Father Randy came by Cedar View Lodge and spoke with my mother. "Lucy said to go ahead and get the moving van lined up and wanted to know what time you will be here tomorrow." I said a silent prayer of thanks for the pastor's help.

Becky had to go through Atkinson on other business today, so she stopped and gave Mom a bottle of Scotch from the stash I'd found in my parents' basement when we cleaned out their house. When Becky got home, she said, "Your mom complained about you the whole time. You probably shouldn't be around during the move tomorrow. Garrett and I can handle it just fine."

I'm thankful that Deputy Garrett agreed to help. He'll drive her to O'Neill and check her into the Four Seasons Nursing Home. I've already signed the papers. Becky said she'd help me move some of Mom's possessions to her new place, and Barry and I will take the rest of it back to Bassett. Boy, have we done a lot of 'stuff moving' lately!

**Tuesday, May 19, 2015:** I could tell from my mother's behavior that moving day felt traumatic for her—and it did for me, as well. Deputy Garrett arrived in the morning and escorted Mom from Atkinson to O'Neill without incident. I felt like a Peeping Tom, watching them from my hiding spot in the parking lot. Initially, Mom didn't realize that her new home is in a locked Alzheimer's unit. Garrett told me later that she had a fit when she found out.

Becky helped move enough of my mother's belongings to the new location to get her by until Barry and I can transport the rest. She said that Mom had a couple of tantrums, so the nurse gave my mother some of her Scotch to calm her down. It's a good thing I signed that elixir over to them.

I am, according to staff experienced in these things, a 'trigger' who sets my mother off, so I managed to stay out of her sight all day as we got Mom and her possessions moved. Afterwards, Barry and I loaded up my car and his truck with items that won't fit into her new room, and we took as much as we could back to Bassett.

**Wednesday, May 20, 2015:** I took the afternoon off work and went to Cedar View Lodge to pack up my mother's remaining items—some to move to O'Neill and the rest to go to storage at our house.

One of the nursing home aides told me that Mom is upset about not having her wardrobe, so I emptied out that bulky piece of furniture and loaded the contents into my car. Barry planned to come help me after work, so I left a note asking him to bring the wardrobe itself in his truck. I drove to the nursing home and brought in a few boxes, leaving them in the hallway for Barry to deliver to her room when he arrived. Coming in with arms full, I rounded a corner and saw Mom coming straight at me— she'd escaped the locked door and marched toward the nurses' desk, obviously in quite a stew. She didn't see me, so I ducked and ran for cover. I hid until a couple of aides got her corralled. Barry arrived with the wardrobe and brought in the boxes. That calmed her down.

Barry and I went back to Cedar View Lodge and loaded his truck and my car with more of Mom's belongings. We got home late, and I saw a couple of calls from the nursing home on caller ID, so I dialed them.

The nurse reported to me that another resident in the Alzheimer's unit had wandered into my mother's room and lay down on her bed. Mom came unglued and hit the woman, hurting her, and she also hit the aide who came to the woman's rescue.

When one resident assaults another, staff is required to report it to the state, so it looks like Mom may have to move again. I told the nurse that I can't handle my mother.

"We know that," she said, "and your mother would be as much of a danger to you as she is to others. We will contact the Avera McKennan Behavioral Health Center in Sioux Falls, South Dakota, and get back to you."

*Good Lord.*

# 22 SUBTERFUGE IN SIOUX FALLS

**Thursday, May 21, 2015:** I took the afternoon off and went to Cedar View Lodge to finish packing Mom's stuff. Barry joined me when he got off work, and we managed to get everything remaining into our two vehicles. I signed the exit paperwork. While we were there, the Four Seasons Nursing Home administrator phoned to tell me they are still deciding whether or not to keep my mother. She asked me some questions about Mom's background and said they should make a decision by tomorrow.

**Friday, May 22, 2015:** I learned that today the Four Seasons Nursing Home staff told my mother she'd be going for a drive in the country. Instead, they took her to the McKennan Behavioral Health Center in Sioux Falls, South Dakota. When they arrived, Mom went to the restroom, and while she attended to that business, the Four Seasons driver left to return to O'Neill.

My mother had an immediate meltdown, and the McKennan staff reported that attempts to calm her were futile. They declared a 'psychiatric emergency' in order to restrain her and administer an antipsychotic injection against her will. The doctor noted that this helped, but the agitation and aggressive behaviors returned soon thereafter.

"The driver brought some of Lucy's clothes and toiletries," the nurse told me. "She'll be okay until after the holiday weekend, when our regular doctor will see her. We think it would be best if you don't visit her, so we'll need you to answer some questions and provide the necessary consents over the phone."

I'm relieved that Mom is finally in professional hands.

**Monday, May 25, 2015:** Memorial Day weekend provided a much-needed bit of fun. Some friends of the family met us at Sunflower Meadows to visit my father. Barry and I brought Terry along, and both she and Dad seemed to enjoy the social occasion.

When we got home, I returned a call from the McKennan Behavioral Health Center. The duty nurse told me my mother had several episodes of violence and agitation and, finally, they sedated her. She put Mom on the phone. Although she asked me about Dad, my mother seemed primarily concerned about her belongings, which I assured her were safe.

Mom called me again a few hours later. She remained fairly calm, but seemed to have forgotten everything we'd talked about earlier. She said she was very worried because she doesn't have any slippers. When I asked the nurse to get her some socks, I mentioned that more than one call per day would likely be counterproductive.

I spent the rest of the holiday weekend catching up on paperwork, paying bills, and tending to neglected chores. I can't even begin to describe how great it felt to do something mundane.

I told Barry I just didn't think I'd be able to do a garden this year, so he and his mom surprised me by putting in spuds, onions, Swiss chard, and green beans. They're my heroes! It's hard to imagine a year without our beloved garden. Planting on Memorial Day provided a bonus—we missed all of the late frosts.

# 23 STABILIZATION

**Thursday, June 3, 2015:** Sue, the social worker at the McKennan Behavioral Health Center, emailed me a letter describing my mother's diagnosis, and she told me to expect a phone call from the geriatric psychiatrist, Dr. Klein. The memo included this information:

"Lucy's most likely diagnosis is Major Neurocognitive Disorder, Alzheimer's Disease Probable, with Behavioral Disturbance. This dementia is neurodegenerative, causing brain cells to develop abnormalities or die. The hallmark of this is memory loss. It also affects the ability to use and understand language, visual-spatial distortions in perception, a decline in executive functions (ability to make and execute a plan), apraxia (impaired ability to carry out motor activities despite intact motor function), and agnosia (failure to recognize objects or people). Many patients also display other psychological and behavioral problems, including agitation and aggression.

"Alzheimer's is, as are all dementias, an untreatable disease for which there is no FDA-approved treatment. Lucy has significant behavioral disturbances associated with this. Antipsychotics are recommended, though they have many dangerous side effects. Unfortunately, the disease, and her conduct, will progress and worsen. Her ability to comprehend and make reasonable decisions will continue to decline."

Dr. Klein telephoned me shortly after I read the diagnosis. He re-emphasized that my mom is not going to get any better.

"We've been treating your mother with an antipsychotic, Zyprexa (olanzapine), which made a bit of improvement in her aggression and uncontrolled agitation. But she remains perseverative regarding her desire to have her purse and medications in her possession. Our staff discusses this with Lucy multiple times each day. Often, she argues and becomes antagonistic with our employees over seemingly endless requests she makes of them, and she can't easily be redirected. Your mother demands a bag to pack up her belongings and tells us that you are coming to pick her up. At times she wanders the unit out of frustration, and during all of these episodes her distress is evident."

Dr. Klein requested my permission to change Mom's prescription to a more potent antipsychotic, Risperdal (risperidone). He said my mother meets the criteria (over sixty-five, aggression, dementia) that require a doctor to give the family a warning that this drug has a slight (3%) risk of death.

"What are the alternatives?" I asked.

"Some families have decided against using it. They had to come and pick up the patient because there was nothing more we could do."

That is not an option for my family, so I consented. I can't handle my mother, and there is no other place that will accept her in her current condition. She is in good physical health. I hope the drug will help, not harm.

**Sunday, June 7, 2015:** I continue to worry about Dad. He seemed groggy and confused when I picked him up this morning at Sunflower Meadows to take him to church. It surprised me, since he'd sounded so good on the phone earlier in the week. I asked Nurse Mardell about it. She thinks his disorientation may be caused by the new prescription he has for stress. She said she will speak to his doctor.

**Wednesday, June 10, 2015:** Penny, the head nurse at McKennan, told me that Mom had a bad episode yesterday. They are still trying to find the right dosage of the new medicine. We talked about the long-term plan, which still is to get her stabilized and placed—in O'Neill, if they will take her back, or somewhere else.

I spent much of the day running around getting financial forms filled out for the upcoming court hearing. Attorney Arganbright asked me the status of the letter he'd requested from Dr. Klein supporting my court petition to obtain guardianship of my mother. I called Sue at McKennan and reminded her we need it before the June 29th hearing. She assured me they are working on it. She also said that if the weekend goes well, the doctor hopes to discharge my mother from their facility next week.

**Thursday, June 11, 2015:** I drove to O'Neill to check on the room that the Four Seasons Nursing Home is holding for my mother. It looked like nothing had been disturbed. I threw away the dead plant in the window and removed some stale snacks from a drawer, so everything will be fresh for her. I felt relieved when Mandy, the social worker, said the nursing home is willing to take Mom back, as long as she is no longer dangerous.

**Monday, June 15, 2015:** I received the letter from Dr. Klein that Attorney Arganbright needs for the upcoming court hearing. In part, it said:

"My recommendations for Lucy include the continued use of an antipsychotic medication for her behaviors. This must be monitored by a physician and the staff at the facility, watching for signs of adverse reactions to the medication or the need to adjust the dosing. She will have to be in a nursing home, as opposed to a facility with a lesser level of care. Lucy should not be driving for a multitude of reasons related to the disabilities imposed by the disease. She does not have the capacity to make her own medical and financial decisions and therefore should have a designated individual making them for her. I reiterate that her present condition is not temporary.

"I support Mrs. Benson's request to obtain legal guardianship of her mother. Some physicians will not proceed with specialized care simply on the authority of a Power of Attorney, but require the consent of a legal guardian. Lucy is argumentative and will not likely agree with all directives made by a POA even when they are in her best interest."

**Tuesday, June 16, 2015:** The McKennan social worker told me the doctor believes the dosage is now correct for the new medication. "The Risperdal seems to produce the calm and relief from distress we've been seeking, and she's doing well with it. We're releasing your mother back to the nursing home in O'Neill tomorrow. We recommend that you do not see her just yet."

The Four Seasons Nursing Home will send their driver to Sioux Falls to pick up Mom, which will work well. But if I'm not supposed to see her, how will I get her to court for the June 29th guardianship hearing? That requires a two-plus hour drive each way between Valentine and O'Neill. I checked with the attorney, and he said not to worry; the information in the doctor's letter should provide ample justification for not bringing her to court.

**Friday, June 19, 2015:** I phoned the Four Seasons Nursing Home to check on my mother. The social worker, Mandy, confirmed that the new drug is doing a pretty good job of taming Mom's anger and aggression, and she transferred my call to the Alzheimer's unit. The duty nurse told me that because my mother still thinks I'm coming to take her home, any visits at this point would likely be unwise. She did say it might be okay to talk, though, and she put me on hold. After a few minutes, my mother picked up the handset.

"Sandy? Sandy?" Mom's voice quivered, and I found it nearly unrecognizable. She asked me repeatedly when I'd be there to pick her up and take her home.

I didn't know how to answer. I think I said something about waiting until her doctor felt confident in her new medication.

*What have I done to her?*

# 24 FATHER'S DAY

**Sunday, June 21, 2015:** Father's Day. My father spent the weekend with Barry and me. Although he seemed less confused than last time I saw him, it is obvious he is not thriving at Sunflower Meadows. Dad asked us to move him closer to our home so he can see us more often. After lunch, I took him to look at both Sandhills Haven in Stuart and Cedar View Lodge in Atkinson, where my mother's former apartment is still open.

Dad remembered that he and Mom visited both places last winter. He still thinks Sandhills Haven is "too institutional and sterile," but he really likes the homey atmosphere at Cedar View Lodge. I told Julie, the administrator, that we'll take the room. She said we can get all of the paperwork completed this week so I can move him next Saturday. I arranged for Mike the Mover to help us again.

**Monday, June 22, 2015:** Mandy, the social worker from the Four Seasons Nursing Home, emailed me: "Just wanted to let you know that your mother expected you to show up this morning. The nurse said that yesterday Lucy wanted to call you every ten minutes, so she finally told her that you were coming tomorrow. This morning, she acted upset and worried because you weren't here. I told her you were probably at work, and she said that you don't work on Saturdays. I reminded her today is Monday. Lucy said you don't like to drive in the afternoon, so she seemed sure that was wrong. We tried to distract her all day, but she is still worried about you."

I feel uncomfortable about them telling Mom all these made-up stories. I asked Mandy if she thought it would be okay for me to visit. She said they'd prefer if I wait until my mother readjusts to her surroundings.

A nurse will perform Dad's assessment at Cedar View Lodge tomorrow. Dr. Grant will administer a physical exam. Julie, the administrator, promised to be there to check my father in when we move him Saturday.

Both Barry and I entirely forgot that today is our wedding anniversary. His mother remembered, though. She gave us a sweet card and fixed us a special dinner. Terry is a real peach. Despite her own health issues, she somehow keeps us grounded.

**Thursday, June 25, 2015:** Dad called early, shaken by a nightmare, he said. He seemed confused, saying my mother is stalking him again, and he'd seen her in his apartment. I reassured him that she can no longer leave O'Neill because she is in a locked wing at the nursing home. Dad said he understands that he had a hallucination, but he is still afraid of her. I hope that moving him from the place they shared an apartment will help him get rid of that ghost.

**Saturday, June 27, 2015:** Another move is safely behind us. I spent yesterday at Sunflower Meadows, where I completed the exit paperwork and settled up with them financially. My father helped me sort out what he will need for his small room at Cedar View Lodge, and I boxed up the rest of it. I took Dad home with me for the night.

Late this afternoon, Mike the Mover cleared everything out of Dad's apartment and drove to our house, where we unloaded items not destined for Cedar View Lodge. Barry is burned out from all the moving, so he begged off this time, knowing we were in excellent hands.

My father and I followed Mike to Atkinson, where he once again expertly unloaded at Cedar View Lodge. Julie navigated Dad through the check-in paperwork and then I took him out for supper. Afterwards, I helped him unpack and get settled into his new apartment. We finished by nine p.m. I put him to bed and tiptoed out of the room to the sound of his snores.

**Monday, June 29, 2015:** Dad and I went to court again today. The judge granted me permanent guardianship of Mom. Following our attorney's instructions, we spent the balance of the day making the necessary changes to my parents' bank and investment accounts and their insurance policies. Although I have a Power of Attorney for my father, Warren thought it best that Dad do all of the signing himself. Our last stop was at my parents' lawyer's office in Bassett, where Dad signed his updated POA and insurance papers. He looked pretty beat by the time we were done, and when we stood to leave, he nearly fell over. It took both the attorney and his secretary to help me get him to my car. He fell asleep on the way back to Cedar View Lodge.

# 25 FAILURE TO THRIVE

**Thursday, July 9, 2015:** We are taking care of some 'deferred maintenance' relating to my father's health. The last several months have been so wild that some things fell between the cracks. Dad had a tumor removed from his leg Monday at the hospital in Atkinson. He told me he'd been watching it grow, but only now that his life is settling down a bit, did he feel comfortable attending to it. He will have a follow-up appointment when the biopsy results come back. He's also having problems with his feet, so we scheduled a date for him with the podiatrist. But I'm actually more worried about his mental health.

Julie, the Cedar View Lodge administrator, called me around eight a.m. "We had quite a time with your father today. He woke up at two-thirty this morning and went to the kitchen for breakfast. He claimed he needed to hurry and eat because of his appointment, which isn't until this afternoon.

"The staff went into his room and saw he'd changed all of his clocks back; he told them it is because of daylight savings. So, they fixed his clocks. Then he went out again and got very irritated when he couldn't get breakfast. They explained they don't serve until seven-fifteen, and it was only five a.m. I hope this afternoon's shot will help."

Cripes! Dad never behaved like this before. Since leaving Sunflower Meadows, though, he's had a lot of issues with telling time. I'm not sure what causes that, or how to fix it. Lately, he sleeps a lot during the day, which may be messing up his perceptions. Also, his room is kind of dark. I think if he can restrict himself to just an afternoon nap, he will be better able to sleep through the night.

After work, Barry and I visited Dad. He'd been messing with his clocks again, so I reset them and reminded him that we stay on daylight savings time until fall. I noticed he has three clocks in the one-room apartment. I asked him if I could have one of them, and he let me take it. I suggested he participate in some of the social and recreational activities Cedar View Lodge offers, instead of sleeping so much.

**Friday, July 10, 2015:** It's hard to believe it's been a year since this adventure in dementia began. I can't help but wonder where we are heading from here. After work, I listened to a message from my mother on our answering machine. No mention of my birthday; she just asked me to come pick her up. Of course, I never expected her to remember, but it's the first time this has ever happened, and I feel a little sad.

I called Four Seasons and asked Mom's nurse if I can visit yet. She said no, they will let me know when they feel it is safe to do so. I asked to speak with my mother, but they said she was sleeping.

**Thursday, July 16, 2015:** The new medication Dr. Grant prescribed to calm my father's increasing anxiety does not appear to be doing the job. I got this email from Julie: "Today when housekeeping came into George's room, they found a pair of cut up underwear in his wastebasket. He also had a pair of jeans in his trash, but she just moved them to his laundry hamper. Do you want to take his scissors from his room on Saturday? Do you want to set up another appointment with Dr. Grant regarding his hallucinations?"

We scheduled the earliest appointment slot available, Monday morning. Julie will transport my father to the office, and I'll phone Dr. Grant afterwards. Julie and I agreed not to tell Dad about it until Monday so he doesn't worry and get himself all worked up. I will visit him Saturday, pick up the scissors, and check on his clothing situation.

**Tuesday, July 21, 2015:** Since my father has been at Cedar View Lodge, his health has taken a nose dive. He has fallen several times, but no broken bones—just bruises. He continues to spend his days in his PJs in bed, in a darkened room, and has to be reminded to come out for meals. Julie said he has no concept of whether it is day or night. The staff continues to complain about his wandering down to the dining room in the wee hours, demanding breakfast.

Dad has hallucinations in which several people live in his room with him. At first, he said it is my mother and me. "Your mom just sits there crocheting, not saying anything. Are you sure that she is locked up and can't be here? I just *know* she is stalking me again." Poor man.

More recently, he told me he's been seeing three children and a six-foot man in his room. He said the children have been doing lots of mischief, like pulling all his clothes out of his drawers and closet, leaving his shoes in the middle of the room where he can trip over them, and cutting up a perfectly good pair of jeans and some underwear. I've now got his scissors.

My father seems preoccupied with toileting. Yesterday, the Cedar View Lodge housekeeper found him on the floor with his pajama bottoms around his ankles and his adult diaper half off. Concerned about both the fall and his apparent disorientation, staff took him to the hospital. A nurse called me from the emergency room. I hurried to Atkinson, bringing some clothing along in order to get him back to the apartment decently.

Today he is scheduled for another functional assessment, and I'm pretty sure he will no longer be considered capable of remaining in assisted living. I've talked to him about moving into the Long-Term Care section of the Bassett hospital. He is willing to go there, but there are no openings; he is on the waiting list. I called Sandhills Haven in Stuart this morning. Their social worker told me they have an opening and can take him immediately. I drove to the facility and filled out the paperwork. Dad said before that he doesn't like that place, so I'm worried.

**Thursday, July 23, 2015:** Barry and I have lost track of how many times we have moved my parents this year. Dad's functional assessment at Cedar View Lodge Tuesday ended up as I'd predicted, and we got him moved and settled into the nursing home section of Sandhills Haven. We cleared the rest of his belongings out of Cedar View Lodge, and I took care of his exit paperwork. Julie said she hopes my father adjusts well to the move, and she asked for his address so staff could send him a card to wish him well.

Sandhills Haven seems to be the right choice for Dad. The aides take excellent care of him, so Barry and I decided to take a much-needed break. We leave first thing in the morning on a three-day camping weekend to celebrate Barry's birthday. His mom volunteered to watch our house.

**Thursday, July 30, 2015:** The mini-vacation worked wonders for Barry and me. We both feel much less stressed. Although I am sorry that my parents are in nursing homes, it is really a relief to come home and enjoy at least some semblance of normal life.

Today I completed the state-mandated guardianship training course I need to handle my mother's affairs. The department will mail me my completion certificate, which our attorney will file with the court.

# 26 A LITTLE BREATHER

**Monday, August 24, 2015:** Life is finally settling into a more comfortable routine for Barry and me. I'm getting a bit caught up at work, and last week I attended, without worry, our summer forestry meeting at Chadron State Park, in the Nebraska Panhandle. What a beautiful site!

Barry took his mother to Fort Robinson State Park this past weekend, as a late 80th birthday gift. They both enjoyed the getaway, staying in a cabin at the historic military outpost. In three weeks, she'll be going home to Florida, and Barry said he regrets that during this crazy summer he hasn't been able to spend much quality time with her.

I stayed home, tending to chores and visiting my parents at their respective nursing homes—yes, the Four Seasons Nursing Home in O'Neill finally okayed in-person visits with my mother.

Mom greeted me by name when I entered her room. I sat in the only chair, and she sat on the edge of her bed. We didn't find much to talk about. She seemed sleepy and unnaturally quiet—undoubtedly under the influence of the anti-psychotic medication. I found that unsettling instead of comforting. After a short, unsatisfying visit, I left her, napping.

I spoke with one of the Alzheimer's unit aides, who filled me in on my mother's new life. "When Lucy first came back here from Sioux Falls, she spent most of her time pacing the hallway, often trying to escape through the locked door when it opened to let someone in or out."

The aide chuckled. "The woman who lives in the room across from your mother sometimes joins her in walking the halls. Once, while Lucy punched numbers into the door lock—I'll bet she had no idea that she came very close to actually figuring that out—her friend came up behind her to watch. Your mom asked, 'what's the code for this door?' and her partner-in-crime said, 'Honey, if I knew that, we'd ALL be outta here!'"

On my way out, I stopped at the nursing station. The duty nurse said my mother is mostly quiet and cooperative now. I'm relieved, but somehow that makes me sad.

**Monday, September 7, 2015:** I visited Dad on Saturday and Mom today, since I'm off for Labor Day. Everything seemed about the same, so I'm hoping things have finally settled down for our family. I arrived home in time to help Terry make a salad, while Barry grilled burgers on the back deck. It felt good to kick back and enjoy a pleasant evening.

**Thursday, September 10, 2015:** The tumor on my father's leg is growing back. Lab tests revealed quickly-progressing skin cancer, but because he is ninety-one years old, the doctor said we can't be too aggressive with treatment—because it might kill him. So, at least for now, we are doing nothing about it.

Dad remains in good spirits, but he is mixed up a lot. Dr. Grant says he has vascular dementia, caused by a series of mini strokes. He usually recognizes me, but sometimes he confuses me with Mom. The social worker at Sandhills Haven told me that, due to his dementia, they will be moving my father into the Alzheimer's wing, possibly as early as next week. The aides there tell me Dad is a joy to be around. I'm grateful to them for caring for him so well.

**Saturday, September 12, 2015:** Yesterday, my mother's nurse told me the doctor is going to reduce the dosage on Mom's anti-psychotic medication. Initially, I felt relief because she seemed like such a zombie when I last visited—just a ghost of her former self. As I think about it more, however, it scares me.

Now that it's too late to really help us, I'm discovering a few resources, like the *Alzheimer's Reading Room* website, that I wish I'd known about from the beginning. Someday I should write a book about all of this and include a list of references for others just beginning their journey through dementia.

A friend of mine, Jill, who is caring for her own elderly parents, wrote, "We daughters perform like Olympians trying to meet all our aging parents' needs and then lie awake at night, trying to resolve the unresolvable situations our parents face. These are scary, depressing, and uncharted waters, with moments of sweetness, bitter-sweetness, and gut punches that are so surreal we can barely think straight."

# PART THREE

## 27 LIFE FLIGHT

**Tuesday, September 15, 2015:** Yesterday morning, I stopped by my mother-in-law's house to say goodbye and wish her safe travels on her journey home to Florida. She smiled and gave me a hug. Something didn't seem quite right, but I couldn't put my finger on it.

Midmorning, Barry picked her up for the two-and-a-half-hour drive to the airport. He called me about one-thirty p.m. "I don't know what's wrong with my mom. She's acting really strange. We went out for lunch and she spilled her drink, and now her conversation isn't making sense. I can't put her on the plane like this. I'm bringing her home."

When they pulled into the driveway I went out to meet them, not knowing what to expect. Barry seemed worried. Terry sat quietly, looking down at her lap. I opened the door and realized the truck seat, and her pants, were wet. Barry came around to the passenger side and we helped her out of the pickup and into a chair on the front porch. She had trouble speaking, and she couldn't turn her head to the right or move her right arm.

"Barry," I said, "you need to get your mother to the emergency room immediately. I think she's had a stroke. You can get her there faster than if we call an ambulance. I'll tell the hospital in Bassett you're coming."

He put a sheet of plastic over the wet seat, and I helped him get her into the pickup before I ran inside to the telephone.

Barry phoned me an hour and a half later. "She did have a stroke and she isn't doing well. I'll let you know when we learn more."

Just before midnight, a Life-Flight helicopter took Terry to Sanford Medical Center in Sioux Falls, South Dakota, where there is a trauma unit and specialized medical staff. Barry hurried home. We grabbed a couple of hours of sleep before leaving at dawn to make the four-hour drive to Sanford.

We found Barry's mother in the critical care unit, unconscious and on oxygen. The doctor told us, "Don't get your hopes up."

Around supper time, a nurse suggested we find a place to stay. "We don't think anything will change overnight." So here we sit in a motel room, worrying and waiting.

**Thursday, September 17, 2015:** In the morning, Terry's status remained the same. The doctor said, "We may be in for the long haul."

Barry brought me home late yesterday so I can tend to our other responsibilities. Tomorrow he will return to Sioux Falls.

Barry said he is scared for her, and I am, too. Things might have been different if we'd recognized the symptoms sooner. We missed that narrow window of time when sometimes patients can be treated to minimize damage from a stroke.

**Thursday, September 24, 2015:** Barry came home on Tuesday. He said, "Mom's still in the critical care unit, but has regained consciousness and her condition is gradually improving. Although she's unable to swallow, she is responding to physical therapy. My mother knows where she is and why she is there. The staff at Sanford is wonderful."

Once Terry's feeding tube is out and she can leave critical care, we will see about transferring her somewhere closer to us. At this point we are not going to even consider trying to get her home to Florida. We are thankful her brother, Kenny, who lives near her house there, has been forwarding her mail and taking care of her yard all summer and will just continue to do so. Ever since Barry's dad died about ten years ago, Kenny has been good about tending to things in Florida for his sister every summer when she visits us.

Barry leaves first thing tomorrow morning to return to Sioux Falls. I have my hands full here.

I'm in packing mode once again. This time we have to move our forestry office to a new building across town. All the practice I've had this year is making packing a snap, and Barry and I have lots of boxes to donate to the cause. Moving day is one week from today.

# 28 MELANOMA

**Friday, October 2, 2015:** I picked up my father at Sandhills Haven and drove him two and a half hours to the dermatologist in Norfolk. The physician excised seven nasty-looking skin cancers from Dad's scalp, left leg, and back, but not the one near his right ankle that he went there to have removed. That one is huge, and the doctor deems it inoperable for a ninety-one-year-old. He said it is the kind of tumor that usually has good results with radiation, and his office made an appointment for Dad with a nearby oncologist. Soon, he should be able to start the regimen.

The treatment sessions may be daily or several times weekly, but we won't know about the schedule until Wednesday. I am unable to handle the special care Dad needs, so I can't stay overnight with him at a motel in Norfolk between treatments. I will have to take him back and forth from the nursing home.

Although my father seems to fully understand what he is up against, he's been surprisingly upbeat. He even insisted on stopping for ice cream on our way back to Sandhills Haven.

I wish we had known, years ago, what we now know about the effects of sunbathing on the human body.

**Wednesday, October 7, 2015:** Gad, what a day! I got up at 'oh-dark-thirty' and picked up my father and the sack lunch the nursing home staff packed for him. When we arrived at the clinic in Norfolk, we learned that this wasn't the first session after all—just an evaluation. Starting October nineteenth, Dad will receive daily treatments, Monday through Friday for four weeks. That's a two-and-a-half hour drive each way for a three-minute appointment—times five days, times four weeks equals a hundred hours of travel for sixty minutes of radiation. Crap, crap, crap.

I'm looking into finding a temporary nursing home placement for my father in Norfolk during that time because I can't transport him and keep my job. More importantly, that much traveling would just be too hard on Dad. Quadruple crap!

And—icing on the cake—when I got home tonight Barry said, "I just found out that Mom can't be treated at our local hospital after she is discharged from Sioux Falls. Monday we'll have to move her to Lincoln for city-sized physical therapy."

Father Randy says that the Lord won't give us more than we can handle. Is God testing us? As my friend, Jill, told me, this situation is CRISIS, all capital letters, and only a monsoon of miracles is going to make this work.

Jill said, "The crazy part is knowing that the medically needy ones are very much at the end of their life span. Calling hospice and settling for quality over quantity makes such good sense, and yet it also seems unimaginable."

I agree. It *is* so hard. As long as my dad and Barry's mom have some spunk, which they do, I can't imagine doing anything to make what life they have left any less hopeful. Both of them have 'do not resuscitate' orders in place, but they aren't at that point, yet. Dad could lose his leg if we don't do the radiation. That won't happen on my watch.

I'm headed to slumberland. I'm a wreck tonight and I have to work tomorrow.

**Friday, October 9, 2015:** Mixed day of good and bad news. The good news is that Valley Grove Care Center in Norfolk will take my father for the duration of the treatments and they will provide the transportation to and from the clinic. The bad news is that the biopsies came back on the seven spots Dad had removed last Friday. Six of them were okay, but the seventh (on his back) is a melanoma and he needs to return so they can make sure they got it all. After I move Dad into Valley Grove next Wednesday, I will stop by the dermatologist's office and make an appointment for that visit. At least today I escaped into the woods for a while to inspect a forestry project, and it really felt good to get some exercise on a beautiful autumn day.

**Monday, October 12, 2015:** A bit of pleasant news: After telling us last week they couldn't do it, Sanford Medical Center transferred Terry to our hospital in Bassett instead of to the facility in Lincoln. My mother-in-law will, after all, be able to receive the physical therapy she needs right here. She continues to improve. Since Barry works at our local hospital, he'll be able to see his mom every day.

**Wednesday, October 14, 2015:** This morning I went to Sandhills Haven and picked up my father, his suitcase, and his meds and took him to Norfolk to check into Valley Grove. Dad was chatty during the drive. "I hope this goes quick—I have a lot to do this week. I've been elected Secretary of State in Alaska. My speech will contain four words: 'Thank you. I quit!'"

I've learned a lot over the past year about dementia, so I just said, "Congratulations!"

I got Dad settled into Valley Grove. His room is huge—a bed, table, a couple of chairs, chest of drawers, and a television set, all separated by an ocean of flooring. The room is so big and empty that it actually echoes when we speak. My father remained cheerful as I showed him how to use the TV remote and adjusted the recliner for him. We ate lunch in the large dining room, sharing a table with a pleasant lady in a wheelchair and a deaf gentleman who smiled at us. I enjoyed watching Dad converse with the woman. Maybe this won't be so bad after all.

On my way out, I stopped by the social worker's office to sign the paperwork. She assured me they would work with the clinic staff to ensure Dad makes it to all of his radiation sessions.

**Thursday, October 15, 2015:** I called my father this morning and asked him how he is doing in his new digs.

"Awful!" he said. "I have nothing to wear and there is going to be a big party tonight. Where is my sport coat?"

"I have it here in my closet. You won't need it for the radiation treatments."

That may have been the wrong thing to say, as he then switched into complaining mode. He said he didn't eat supper last night because he had nobody to sit with. Of course, when I called the nurses' station, they told me he not only ate, but had some great company. Frankly, I'm so exhausted with all of this that I'm just barely staying above water.

# 29 MONEY WORRIES

**Saturday, October 17, 2015:** Tonight, I did some number-crunching to get a handle on how my folks are doing financially—my initial calculations were way off the mark. I based them on the assumption that Mom and Dad would remain together in assisted living for several years. It's too bad my parents sold their house in such a hurry; had they waited until summer—when real estate sells faster in our area—they probably could have netted another $30,000.

To ensure my parents have equal access to the funds needed for their care, the attorney helped split their assets evenly between them when the court granted me guardianship of my mother. Now, I administer a checking and savings account for each of them. Dad receives $1,100 in social security income each month, plus a $900 pension payment; Mom just gets $700 in social security. Their combined expenses are close to $14,000 per month for the nursing homes, plus the copays needed for their medical expenses. This is burning through their savings at lightning speed.

Although I understand that the law is designed to protect the elderly, I believe that the state's financial requirements for guardianship are draconian. If Mom runs out of cash first, we may have to go to court to keep Dad's money for him to live on. We do have a chance to win because of Nebraska's 'spousal impoverishment' law. The bottom line is: when we spend everything, they go on Medicaid.

My friend, Jill, who is dealing with similar parental circumstances, advised me: "When their money is almost spent, put your parents into the best care center in town, because once the funds are gone, the facility must keep the patients when they shift to Medicaid. The scramble is getting them into 'the best' if there is a waiting list."

Jill lives in a large city. I told her, "It's worse in rural areas. The biggest thing I've learned is that Nebraska has no assistance network to provide information for families. The social workers at the nursing homes have been the most help. I did have Dad in the best nursing home in our area, but had to move him out for the radiation treatments. I'm hoping there will still be an opening there when he's done, since we can't afford to hold his room while paying for his stay in Norfolk."

**Sunday, October 18, 2015:** While I visited my father at Valley Grove this afternoon, he acted quite agitated. I had to explain again to him why he is there. We walked down the hall to give him some exercise. When we returned to his room, he stopped in front of the nameplate on his door and frowned. "I don't want everyone to know I'm in this room. Can you take my name off?"

"I'll ask the nurse about it, Dad. I think they need it so they can find you. There are a lot of patients here."

Both of my parents have what's called 'Sundowners Syndrome,' in which their daily behavior worsens starting in the late afternoon. For Dad, that is when he becomes most confused and upset. In Mom's case, that's the time she gets particularly aggressive and angry. Although this is a well-documented phenomenon common to dementia patients, I've been unable to find any information about how to deal with it, other than employing techniques such as reducing noise.

**Monday, October 19, 2015:** The doctor drew 'targets' on my father's leg today; the first radiation session is tomorrow.

Cindy, the social worker at Valley Grove said, "Changing residences has been difficult for your dad, but we want to work with him and try to get him into a routine. Your father had an issue today. He went into the bathroom on his own, instead of paging us, as he is supposed to do. An aide found him on the floor with his pants around his ankles, lying in a puddle of urine and feces."

Cindy said the fall didn't hurt him, and they cleaned him up, but I worry and worry. And worry some more.

**Tuesday, October 20, 2015:** Terry's Medicare-paid stay at the Bassett hospital ran out. Today an ambulance transported her to Sandhills Haven, the nursing home in Stuart that housed my dad until he went to Valley Grove in Norfolk.

Barry oversaw the move and said it went well. "Stuart is only a half-hour away, so I can still visit her daily."

My mother-in-law has incurred some huge medical expenses. The helicopter transport company billed over $60,000 for the flight from Bassett to Sioux Falls, and we don't yet know if Medicare will cover that.

When I got home tonight after a particularly tough day at work, I returned a call from Jane, a nurse at Valley Grove. "George fell again today, but has no injuries. He asked why he is here."

Dad told me last Sunday that he understands that he is in Norfolk for treatments. He may need to be reminded.

Our recent experiences with eldercare have inspired Barry and me to purchase long-term care insurance for ourselves. We have scheduled an appointment for a representative from a nationally-known company to administer cognitive tests to us. If we pass those, and our physical exams, we will qualify. It isn't cheap, but our eyes are now open to just how expensive old age can become.

**Thursday, October 22, 2015:** Cindy at Valley Grove said, "We moved your father closer to the nurse's station, and it went very well. George found the room more appropriate for him; he said he didn't need all that space in the other room. He is a little tired from his treatment today. He is such a gentleman—he is so polite and always says 'please' and 'thank you.'"

**Friday, October 23, 2015:** This evening I chatted with my friend, Jill. We're both wrestling with parental 'quantity vs. quality' of life issues. We joked about taking up smoking and drinking so we would die younger, but happier.

I said, "I struggle daily with the guilt I feel for putting my parents 'in prison'—but, left on their own, they would hurt themselves, each other, or someone else."

"My dad constantly refers to their lovely senior apartment complex as prison," Jill said. "I've been advised to settle them into assisted living now, while they still have some health and brains so they can bond with caretakers. We're looking. Right now we are doing in-home care for twenty dollars an hour. Four hours a day, seven days a week, plus rent/utilities/groceries makes the total cost roughly the same as assisted living."

"It sounds like the in-home help is great for your parents. Staying in their house can give them a sense of security and I think it can help keep them lucid longer. We've moved my mom and dad ten times in ten months. Since you don't have the danger of one parent abusing the other, in-home help is certainly a cheaper option than having two in separate nursing homes. Based on our experience, I have my doubts about the value of assisted living. The facilities around here seem to want perfect tenants."

# 30 THE CONSEQUENCES OF WANDERING

**Sunday, October 25, 2015:** Today featured an upbeat visit with my father. He likes his new room, and I'm happy that the better location makes it easier for the employees to keep an eye on him. The dining room, all decked out for Halloween, felt cheery. Dad seems to have made friends with quite a few of the residents, and he mixes well with the group.

**Wednesday, October 28, 2015:** Cindy at Valley Grove said, "We had trick n' treat here for the staff's children and residents' grandchildren. Your father liked seeing all the little ones. He enjoys looking nice. Every morning he makes sure he gets his hair combed just right and shirt tucked in. He is becoming very dear to us! We all answer his questions and redirect as needed."

**Saturday, October 31, 2015:** I spent Halloween on the road. I drove three hours to Norfolk for lunch with Dad, and I'm not sure he even remembered me. That seems incongruent with what Cindy told me Wednesday about how well he's been doing.

On my way home, I dropped in to see Mom at the nursing home in O'Neill, and she isn't in very good shape either—but she looked at me, so I think she knew she had company. From there, I went to Sandhills Haven in Stuart to visit my mother-in-law. She recognized me, but cried in seeming frustration at what the stroke has done to her body.

**Monday, November 2, 2015:** The head nurse at Valley Grove told me that Dad has been walking into other residents' rooms, so the facility can no longer keep him. He still has eleven radiation sessions to go, or about two weeks' worth. I'm trying to figure out what to do.

My friend, Jill, sounded incensed when I told her about my father's pending eviction. "Can't that nursing home manage anything at all, especially for a short-term medical crisis? A few more treatments and he likely will be happy to stay put and nap anyway. Have you contacted your state representative about your ongoing struggles? States have to step up on this elder care issue. And it will take some yelling before that happens."

**Tuesday, November 3, 2015:** The nursing homes all have monthly 'family meetings,' where employees update patients' adult children on their parent's care. Cindy, the social worker at Valley Grove, emailed me the agenda for this afternoon's conference call. She apparently isn't in the loop about the new crisis. "The meeting will consist of an overview of George's care: staff from dietary, activities, social services, and nursing will report their involvement with George since he has been here. We'll review the care he is receiving and how well he is adjusting to his new environment. We will report his current medical status and where he is with his treatments. Just ask any questions you may have. We understand this has to be very difficult for you."

My reply: "Thank you, Cindy. I got a call from your facility yesterday advising me that, due to my father's habit of going into other people's rooms, Valley Grove will be unable to keep him for the duration of his treatments. The nurse suggested we discontinue the regimen and move him out. However, the oncologist told me that without the radiation, Dad is likely to lose his leg, and I don't want to do that to him.

"The nurse said we can hire someone to be with my father 24/7, but financially that is impossible for us. I am unable to stay with him myself or transport him for five hours daily, because I don't have enough vacation time. I can't afford to quit my job because we need the income in order to live. My husband has nearly exhausted his work leave, due to his mother's recent stroke and ongoing major medical issues. I have no siblings or other relatives to help us with this. I don't know what to do."

After the afternoon conference call, Cindy contacted other nursing homes in the area to check for openings, and then she phoned me. No male beds are presently open in Norfolk."

I said, "I spoke with a physician's assistant who saw Dad today, and she is willing to work with some medications to get the wandering in check. She will be calling you soon."

**Wednesday, November 4, 2015:** Early today, Cindy reported: "George had a good night. We put alarms on him so we know when he gets up. He used his call light when he had to go to the bathroom."

I spent the morning on the phone with three of my father's doctors and two nursing homes. All of the doctors and the social worker at Sandhills Haven told me they think the staff at Valley Grove is being unreasonable. Dr. Torres, the oncologist, said Dad's overall condition is more age-linked than cancer-related. The doctor agrees that it will be best to expedite treatment and get him back to familiar surroundings. He said my father is showing good response to the radiation, and he will increase the daily dosage to shorten the remaining nine treatments to six. This means I can bring him back to Sandhills Haven at the end of next week. Somehow, I managed to shame the nursing home into going along with this plan

It is also fortunate for our family that Sandhills Haven will take my father back. Due to a nurse shortage, new admissions are shut down until they can hire someone to replace an RN who quit. But the social worker told me they will readmit Dad.

Later, Cindy from Valley Grove got back to me. "Our Director of Nursing said that we will make it work for George. I am working on his transition plan for a week from Friday. We will have him packed and the discharge papers ready for your signature."

**Thursday, November 12, 2015:** My father fell again today but, thankfully, he sustained no injuries. I will be really glad to get him back into Sandhills Haven tomorrow. The staff there likes him; they even painted his room during his absence.

Unfortunately, Dad's mobility stinks. He is in a wheelchair all the time now, since the physician's assistant adjusted his meds to reduce his wandering. This means he gets almost no exercise. I'm confident that his favorite nurse at Sandhills Haven will have him back on his walker in no time.

The nurse at Valley Grove said the radiation has not caused my father any pain or discomfort, and it certainly hasn't affected his appetite. Last week, I had to replace all of his jeans with pants a size larger. I'm glad he eats well—there isn't much else he seems to enjoy any more.

My mother-in-law's condition has nosedived, and she seems to be shutting down. Barry spent all day with her, but she isn't responsive. He's home resting tonight, but is having a hard time. He will return to her bedside in the morning.

Barry's mom told him that she doesn't want any heroics when it's time for her to move on. We are fairly certain that, short of a miracle, she won't be recovering from her stroke. Terry is a wonderful woman, always doing for others. The past couple of months must have been the hardest of her life because everything is reversed, and others have been doing for her.

**Friday, November 13, 2015:** What a change in Dad since I saw him last Saturday. Today he seemed almost catatonic. I took him to the Valley

Grove dining room for lunch before bringing him back to Sandhills Haven. He could barely talk, and when I could hear him, I couldn't understand a word he said. He had trouble finding his mouth with his fork, but wouldn't take any help. He just nibbled at his food, and the aide said he'd refused to eat breakfast, too. I wonder if the increased radiation dosage did that to him.

When we got to Sandhills Haven, Dad's favorite nurse met us at the car to help him inside. She looked flabbergasted when she saw him. She said it seemed obvious to her that the Valley Grove staff had drugged my father heavily to keep him from wandering. His feet were bluish, indicating poor circulation resulting from being confined in a wheelchair.

I couldn't believe my eyes at Dad's reaction to seeing his nurse. He absolutely lit up. She said, "It will take a few days, but I think we can get him into better shape again."

My father gobbled down a piece of cake and some ice cream as soon as he got settled into his old room. He grinned from ear to ear. Thank God he is back in a good place.

# 31 AN ANGEL LOST

**Saturday, November 14, 2015:** Terry is unresponsive. The doctor said he is not expecting her to last much longer. I can't figure out how she is hanging on, unable to eat or drink. The staff continues to provide good care, but she is essentially in hospice now.

Barry has been with his mother every day. I offered to spell him, but he said my best function now is to hold things together at home. My husband is amazing.

**Wednesday, November 18, 2015:** Terry died this afternoon. We will sorely miss her. Barry and I were at her side when she passed, and we stayed with her until the funeral home staff came for her. Afterwards, we took a walk in the park next to the nursing home. When we returned, the staff had made up the bed, and a bouquet of flowers sat atop it.

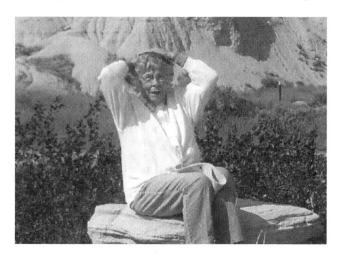

**Thursday, November 19, 2015:** Handling the details after a family member's death is a first for me, but not for Barry, who helped his mother make arrangements after his father passed away a decade ago. There are so many matters to attend to, more than I imagined.

People have already asked us what we plan to do with my mother-in-law's home in Florida. One person even suggested we hire a company to do an estate sale and put the house on the market, without us ever going there. Barry said he thinks that's crazy, and I agree. I've always heard it is best to do nothing until the immediate shock and grief have passed. Uncle Kenny will continue to mow the lawn and forward the mail. The utilities are on auto-pay, so we just need to keep an eye on the bank balance. Once we put Terry to rest, we will figure out when we can go to Florida to settle her estate.

Barry is doing fairly well, all things considered. He said that wrapping up his mother's affairs helps keep his mind occupied. He strung up some Christmas lights on the front porch tonight. We haven't decorated for Christmas in a long time, but we're doing it this year; we even have a little tree. Barry adorned it with the hand-painted ornaments his mother had made for him over the years.

**Monday, November 23, 2015:** Barry and I attended Sandhills Haven's holiday soup-and-pie supper. We ate with my father and his Alzheimer's unit cohorts. Dad displayed fine form and had everyone in stitches.

My father's surgery wounds are healing nicely, much better than anticipated. We canceled his December 16th follow-up appointment. The excision site is completely healed, so Dr. Grant doesn't see any reason to mess with it.

My mother is hanging in there. I got a couple of calls this week from her keepers. They said the nice weather made her think she's ready to 'get outta that joint.' When I phoned her, Mom told me she has some boxes packed and asked me if I know where to find her. I assured her I do but, "Rats, I have to work today and I've used up all of my vacation time." That's the one thing she seems to understand, that I need to work.

**Wednesday, November 25, 2015:** Barry and I really appreciate the employees at Sandhills Haven. Today we brought them a huge fruit and candy basket, with this note:

*Thanksgiving has always been our favorite holiday, and this year we are especially grateful for each and every one of you. You provide an essential service to our community and you do it with compassion and spirit. The Sandhills Haven staff brings 'TLC' to a new level. You demonstrate both expertise and kindness as you gently and professionally tend to our loved ones.*

*Whether you were involved with Terry Benson's end-of-life hospice or are currently caring for George Geib, you are the professional, effective team that makes Sandhills Haven live up to its motto, "Sandhills Haven Has Heart."*

**Friday, November 27, 2015:** What a strange and quiet holiday, with no kinfolks present. Our neighbor Becky invited Barry and me to share a delicious Thanksgiving dinner with her family. I don't know how I'd have survived this past year without her support.

I'm off today, but Barry has to work. When the funeral director called and said he was unable to pick up Terry's ashes at the crematorium in O'Neill, I volunteered to do it. I set off under gloomy, gray skies.

I stopped at the nursing home first, to see my mother. When I told her why I came to town, she didn't seem to remember my mother-in-law, but urged me to get on my way. "It sounds like you have something important to do, so go."

The sun peeked out just before I pulled open the heavy wooden door of the mortuary. It took a moment for my eyes to adjust to the dim light inside. Nobody greeted me. My footsteps echoed as I made my way to the back, where I finally found someone to help me. The man apologized, saying everyone else had the holiday off. He thanked me for coming and handed me the urn.

Outside in the now-brilliant sunshine, I paused to examine the heavy, wood container, beautifully painted as an antique barn. Barry chose it because his mother loved old farmsteads, and she spent many hours photographing, sketching, and painting them. I opened my car door and set the box carefully on the passenger seat.

During that hour-long drive back to Bassett, I found myself repeatedly glancing at the little package, musing that today would be the last time I ever took Terry for a car ride—just the two of us. Without thinking, I found myself talking to her, telling her things I'd meant to say before she passed away—such as what a wonderful mother-in-law she'd been, how much I learned from her, and how much I will miss her.

**Wednesday, December 2, 2015:** Barry delivered the eulogy today at Terry's memorial service; it left not a dry eye in the house. I decided against bringing my mother, but I picked Dad up at Sandhills Haven, and he sat with us in the front pew at the church. He seemed completely in possession of his faculties, and he obviously enjoyed the opportunity to visit with old friends and partake of the delicious luncheon the church ladies prepared.

Terry's ashes now sit on a shelf at our house—awaiting the day we can take them to their final resting place with Barry's father, in upstate New York.

## 32 GOLDEN ANNIVERSARY

**Wednesday, December 30, 2015:** My parents' situation has finally stabilized, and I've fallen into a weekend routine of visiting them. I might be the only person in Nebraska who has the door access codes memorized for the Alzheimer's units in two different nursing homes.

In mid-December, I brought my mother her Christmas card file and some cards. She could only remember a handful of the names, so I helped her address greetings to her sister, brother, and a couple of old friends. Afterwards, I wrote to the others on her list, thinking that otherwise they might wonder why they hadn't heard from my parents.

Christmas Eve afternoon, I gave a couple of little gifts to Mom, and we had a pleasant visit. That evening Barry and I took my father to the early service at our church in Bassett. Dad seemed cheerful and conversed brightly with the parishioners. When I brought him back to Sandhills Haven, I noticed another patient wearing my father's watch. I asked Dad if he knew about that.

"Yes, that's fine. I don't need it."

Only then did I notice my father's wedding ring absent from his finger. I asked his nurse and the aide about it. I'm certain he had it on when he returned from Valley Grove. The aide helped me search his room. We asked Dad if he'd seen it, but he said he didn't know. Remembering his earlier episodes of discarding his clothing, I wondered if he'd thrown it away.

**Friday, January 15, 2016:** My father is recovering well from the radiation and can often converse normally, with only a few lapses into the other world he sometimes lives in. He'll be ninety-two in April. Mom is essentially gone, just inhabiting the shell of an otherwise-healthy eighty-six-year-old body. Sometimes she remembers who I am, other times she doesn't. It's tough to watch, but I'm glad that my parents are in good hands, their basic needs are being met, and that I continue to have opportunities to spend time with them.

Barry and I have been discussing going to Florida in the spring to settle Terry's estate. That depends on things holding stable here, though. We're still taking one day at a time.

**Sunday, February 14, 2016:** We're getting my father out and about a little. Last Sunday, Barry and I 'kidnapped' Dad from Sandhills Haven and took him to the matinee at the theater in Stuart. He seemed to enjoy it.

Today, Valentine's Day, I accompanied my father to Sandhills Haven's ice cream social. He does love his sweets. Although we couldn't bring my mother for today's occasion, I asked Dad what he thinks about having a little get-together with Mom in a couple of weeks to honor their fiftieth wedding anniversary. He agreed.

**Tuesday, February 23, 2016:** I've been working on arrangements for a small party for my parents. Their anniversary is Friday, but we'll celebrate Saturday when Barry and I are off work. The kitchen staff at Sandhills Haven agreed to bake a special cake, and I reserved the facility's recreation room from eleven a.m. until noon. I had to get permission from the nursing home's director to have my mother there, since her restraining order is still in place. I assured him that my mother's aggression is under control and that we will have four competent adults present to supervise. Father Randy and our friend, Chris, offered to bring Mom from O'Neill and take her back to the Four Seasons afterwards. I am keeping my fingers crossed that this plan will succeed.

**Saturday, February 27, 2016:** The party went off without a hitch. My parents seemed surprised and pleased to see each other. They were all smiles for the camera. Mom even reverted to her 'good hostess' manners, offering to package up portions of leftover cake for the guests to take along when leaving.

The festivities must have tired my parents out; by the end of the hour, I noticed both of them nodding off. When I touched her shoulder, my mother said, "Hurry up and get your coat on, George, so we can go home."

Father Randy distracted Mom while I sneaked Dad out of the room. I returned in time to see the priest leading my mother, looking confused, to the car for the ride back to the Four Seasons.

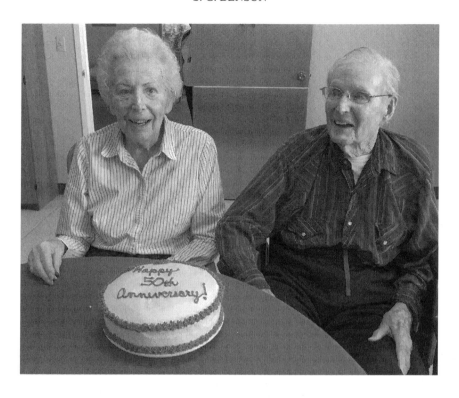

# 33 LAST RITES

**Monday, February 29, 2016:** Returning to the office from a long, cold day in the woods, I found a message on the answering machine from an employee at Sandhills Haven. "Your father is having some health issues; please come to the nursing home after you get off work today."

When I arrived, the nurse told me Dad hasn't been eating, and he may have a urinary tract infection. "Dr. Grant will see him tomorrow, but so far we haven't found anything else out of order."

I found my father seated at the table in the Alzheimer's unit's tiny dining and recreation room. His eyes were closed and his supper sat in front of him, untouched. Looking up from cajoling two other residents to eat, the aide greeted me.

"Dad," I said, taking his hand. "Do you want some supper?"

He opened his eyes and shook his head. I thought he looked extremely tired. He finally took a sip of water, and I wheeled him back to his room. He fell asleep almost immediately.

**Thursday, March 3, 2016:** Tuesday's medical appointment didn't reveal anything new. Dad is continuing to fade. I've visited him after work every day, but he doesn't seem to be present, even though he is conscious. When I talk to him, he just stares into space. The staff told me he hasn't been eating much; mostly he just sleeps. I'm shocked, because it's only been a week since the anniversary party. He acted just fine, then.

His favorite nurse, a veteran of these situations, told me that he may be starting to shut down. "He is exhausted, and he may be ready to move on."

**Saturday, March 5, 2016:** Sandhills Haven's social worker called me late yesterday afternoon. She asked me to come to the nursing home and be prepared to remain for a while. I phoned Father Randy, and he met me there. We entered Dad's room and found him sleeping. His face looked serene; he didn't appear to be experiencing any discomfort. I spoke quietly to him, but he did not respond.

Father Randy and I sat with him for a bit; then we walked out into the hall, where we discussed the next steps as nurses and aides came and went from my father's room. Although I didn't feel hungry, the priest insisted I go get some supper, while he remained at Dad's bedside. When I returned, my father appeared to be the same, but the nurse said his breathing had become shallower.

I held Dad's hand as the priest administered the last rites. Before he left, Father Randy asked if I'd be all right, waiting and watching alone. I said I would.

The world seemed to stand still. I stayed by my father's side, speaking softly to him of fond memories, telling him how much I love him, and praying. Occasionally, I ventured into the hallway to stretch my legs. The building quieted as residents went to bed, leaving aides to thumb through magazines and nurses to attend to paperwork. Every half hour or so, an RN stopped by to check on Dad, shake her head at me, and leave again. My eyes grew heavy, and I nodded off in a chair.

Sometime after midnight, I felt a gentle hand on my shoulder and I opened my eyes.

"It's time," the nurse said.

I reached for my father's hand, but he did not awaken. I could hear his respiration, now ragged and irregular. The nurse stood by, stethoscope in hand, as we watched him take his last breath.

The undertaker handed me some papers before wheeling my dad away. I signed them robotically, then got into my car and drove home, in what felt like a trance.

After getting a few hours of sleep, I drove to O'Neill this morning to tell my mother the news. She stared at me blankly, obviously not comprehending. I feel alone.

**Friday, March 11, 2016:** This week has been a whirlwind of legal notifications and preparations for Dad's memorial service, planned for tomorrow. Both Father Randy and the funeral home have provided a tremendous amount of logistical and emotional support. I don't believe I could have got through this without them.

Barry helped me collect Dad's belongings from the nursing home. After all of the moving we went through with my parents, I found it ironic that Dad's possessions all fit into five boxes.

I telephoned Aunt Marie last Saturday to tell her that her brother passed away; she took the news well. I mentioned to her that years ago

Dad told me he wanted his ashes scattered at sea, but she didn't know anything about that desire. After some research, I learned that California has strict laws against scattering human ashes within twelve nautical miles of the coast, so it may not be possible for us to fulfill that wish. For now, we'll keep my father's ashes on the shelf. Eventually, we will find a resting place for both his ashes and my mother's, when her time comes.

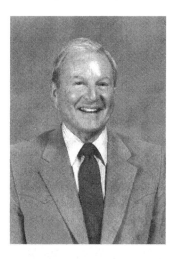

My parents had the foresight to write their own obituaries while they were still cognizant. In their files I even found the photos they wanted to include. My father looked young and vibrant in his picture. All I had to do is add a few finishing touches to his words.

Besides putting the obituary in the local paper, I sent it to the newspapers in Prescott, Arizona, and La Jolla, California, where my parents lived for many years. I also put a brief death notice in the paper in Santa Barbara, California, Dad's birthplace in 1924.

Some of my parents' friends responded to that effort. Barbara, from Arizona, wrote, "Thanks so very much for making sure George's obituary was in the *Courier*. I smiled through my tears as I read about this wonderful friend." And Joan, from La Jolla, asked her daughter to call and thank me.

**Saturday, March 12, 2016:** I drove to O'Neill to pick up my mother for the memorial service. The nursing home staff had done her hair and dressed her nicely. She seemed confused about our destination, but glad to be on an outing. We arrived in Bassett early enough to drive by my parents' old house, but Mom didn't remember it.

About thirty people were at the church; my mother sat in the front row with Barry and me. She seemed to recognize the trappings of a funeral, and several times she asked me who had died. I wrestled with the contradicting advice I'd read about whether or not it is a kindness to only tell Alzheimer's sufferers once that a loved one has died. Older protocol insisted they be told over and over again. Before the service began, I led her to a table in the parish hall where Barry and I had set out photographs of Dad, many of which included her. I told her who had died, but it did not seem to sink in.

Father Randy gave a lovely eulogy. Earlier, he had asked me if I wanted to do a tribute, but I declined, feeling unable to handle it emotionally. Today, my mother kept me busy attending to her needs, which made me glad I wouldn't have to leave her side in order to speak to the congregation.

Mom seemed to enjoy the delicious meal prepared by the church ladies. But as soon as she finished her food, she got up and began looking around the room. Finally, she approached me, just as I ate my last forkful.

"Where's George? I can't find him, and we need to go home."

I struggled to answer her. Several people, who were close enough to hear, looked at us with sadness.

Father Randy came to the rescue. "It looks like the cleanup crew has everything handled, Lucy. Why don't you let Barry take you home? George is okay."

Barry took her back to O'Neill and I went home. It's still early evening, but I've decided to go straight to bed. I feel like I could sleep for a century.

**Monday, March 14, 2016:** Mom turned eighty-seven today. Hallmark card in hand, I visited her after work. Three colorful balloons and a "Birthday Girl" sign graced her door. I found her in the activity room, staring vacantly at a puzzle.

"Happy birthday, Mom," I said, handing her the envelope.

She took it, but her eyes didn't register recognition. "Thank you. Have you seen George?"

# 34 A NEW NORMAL

**Thursday, March 24, 2016:** The certified copies of my father's death certificate arrived in the mail, listing the cause as "Failure to Thrive." I suppose that's the only thing it could be called, since he'd beat his cancer, and nothing showed up during his final doctor's exam. Looking back over the past year and a half, I'm stunned to realize that my mother, who seemed to have the biggest care-need crisis, is the lone survivor of Barry's and my parents.

At least the financial strain should ease. I received a letter from Dad's pension plan administrator, notifying me that under my father's annuity policy, Mom is entitled to receive his monthly pension for the remainder of her life. That, plus only paying for one nursing-home room, should stretch their savings a bit further.

My mother seems to be stable for now, so in the morning Barry and I are leaving for Florida to settle Terry's estate. The social worker at the Four Seasons Nursing Home suggested we wait until we get back, and then bring all of the sympathy cards to Mom at once. That should help her realize that Dad is gone.

**Monday, April 11, 2016:** Barry and I are back from the Sunshine State. That's a *long* drive, two and a half days each way. But we got a lot done while we were there. Not only did we hold a second, well-attended memorial service for my mother-in-law, we got the legal matters handled, and most of Terry's belongings sorted into "keep" and "toss" categories. We performed a ton of maintenance on the house—replaced the shed roof and toilet, did some painting, and repaired some squirrel holes in the house's soffits.

Barry and I breathed a shared sigh of relief as we pulled into our driveway at home yesterday and joked that we'll be glad to get back to our jobs so we can rest.

**Thursday, April 14, 2016:** Dad would have turned ninety-two today. Life just doesn't seem the same without him. I wonder if it ever will.

**Tuesday, April 19, 2016:** My mother seemed pretty much 'out of it' when I went to her nursing home for the monthly family conference. I arrived early, hoping to have a good visit with her, but she didn't seem to know me or want to talk. She lay on her bed with her eyes closed, but her tapping foot suggested she wasn't sleeping. I read to her from her favorite daily devotional book, but even that didn't get her attention.

As I waited for the meeting to begin, I peeked into Mom's dresser drawers, expecting to find neatly folded clothing. Instead, I saw a jumble of wrinkled shirts, mismatched socks, and a stained sweater. The woman who raised me had never tolerated such a mess in *my* drawers, much less her own.

From the table by the window, I picked up a word game booklet dated 2011. Mom taught me to be bold—to do crossword puzzles in ink. These posers featured her tidy printing on the first few pages. Leafing through the magazine, I noticed a transition from ink to pencil. The writing became sloppier and erasure marks increased from one puzzle to the next.

I didn't gain any insight from the family conference. I learned everything I needed to know today from my mother's room.

**Monday, May 16, 2016:** I received a letter from the Veterans' Administration last week regarding benefits that may be available for Mom. Today, I stopped by the Veterans' Service Office to get more information. The clerk said that if we submit the application this year, we can deduct Dad's funeral costs. She also mentioned that Mom should qualify to receive Dad's Social Security payments now, which are higher than her own. I wish I would have known about this earlier. The Social Security Administration must just assume that survivors already know about these things.

I called the Social Security office and found out that Mom qualifies for an additional $714 per month under the Widow's Annuity. She can also get a lump sum of $255 to offset Dad's funeral expenses. The secretary set up an appointment for me with a caseworker at the end of June, which gives me time to round up the documents they'll need. Once the paperwork has been processed, the higher payments will be retroactive to the month of Dad's death.

**Sunday, June 19, 2016:** This is my first Fathers' Day without Dad. I spent a couple of hours looking through old family photos and remembering some fun times. Not only do I miss him; I miss Mom, too, or at least the pre-dementia mother I used to know.

**Sunday, July 10, 2016:** Barry and I visited Mom. Up and about, she seemed pretty chipper. Even though she gave birth to me sixty-two years ago, she no longer knows my name. Barry said, "It's so sad to see her this way." It is, but it has become our 'new normal.'

**Monday, July 18, 2016:** Last week, I received the annual guardianship reporting packet from the county court—with many forms to complete and return by the end of the month. Despite the guardianship/conservator class I took a year ago, I'm still befuddled. I gathered the required documents and dropped them off at our attorney's office. It's worth paying him to ensure it gets done right.

I took Mom to a couple of medical appointments today, and then attended the monthly family meeting at the nursing home. The staff suggested I bring in some of my parents' photo albums. The nurse said that in dementia patients, old memories linger longer than newer ones. She said my mother may recall some of the faces and locations from many years ago. I have a whole bookcase full of their photographs. It's worth a try.

**Saturday, August 27, 2016:** The scrapbook experiment seems to be working. Often, Mom recognizes a person or a setting, even if she can't put a name to it. I found it interesting that she remembered the name of the family dog from her childhood. Each week, I leave an album with her, and then bring another to replace it the following weekend. It's been fun for me to look at the pictures along with her.

I think the nursing home aides enjoy it as much as I do. Today, one of them stopped me in the hall as I headed toward my mother's room with a fresh book. "Your parents sure did a lot of travelling."

I nodded. "And, they took a lot of photos."

"Some of us spend time with your mother, looking at them with her. This week we saw the pictures from your parents' Amazon River cruise." She blushed. "Did you know that there are NAKED people in some of those shots?"

I stifled a laugh. "Yes, the ship took my folks far up the river to a natives' village that white people rarely visited. Most of the youngsters, and even some of the adults, wore little to no clothing. Mom told me afterwards that the children ran up to her and touched her white arms—a skin color they'd never seen."

# 35 UNDER NEW MANAGEMENT

**Sunday, September 18, 2016:** Today, while visiting my mother, I took her into the nursing home's fenced outdoor garden area for some exercise. When she sat to rest on a bench, I examined our surroundings. A few fall flowers were blooming and I noticed that someone has kept the beds weeded and trimmed. A rural-type mailbox with a little red alert flag stood at the edge of the sidewalk, apparently as a decoration, or to allow residents to "check the mail." I opened it and recoiled when I found it full of discarded cigarette butts. This is a non-smoking facility, so I speculated that perhaps employees or visitors come out here to sneak a smoke. When I reported it to the front desk, the attendant rolled her eyes and said, "The new owners can take care of it."

Surprised, I asked for further details, but she just said I'd be getting a letter.

**Monday, October 17, 2016:** I went to court this morning to finish settling my father's affairs. It seemed perfunctory, mostly just to ensure that the county inheritance tax had been paid.

Afterwards, I drove to the Four Seasons for the October family meeting, where a nurse told me that my mother is losing weight. I sat with Mom in the dining room as she ate lunch. She seems to be doing well with the mechanical task of eating. I noticed several other residents were being fed by aides. Mom didn't eat very much. The kitchen staff provides her with extra whole milk and a supplement, but it doesn't seem to be enough.

I received a letter from the nursing home notifying me the facility is changing hands and assuring me that services will continue uninterrupted. I have my doubts, considering the unhappy demeanor I've noticed lately among the employees.

**Friday, November 18, 2016:** The transfer of the Four Seasons Nursing Home to new owners doesn't seem to be going as smoothly as promised. For several weeks I've been trying to get the accounting department to straighten out billing errors resulting from the shift to the new company. I spoke to the office manager, who adjusted last month's invoice and promised she'd fix the problem. I wrote a check for what she said is the correct amount for this month. I then received the November bill for the erroneous amount, so today I drove to O'Neill to discuss it with them in person.

We had about five inches of snow overnight. The highways were clear, but the nursing home's parking lot was a mess—with snow pushed every which way, leaving few parking spaces accessible. It looked like the plow had damaged the curbs; little bits of concrete were scattered about. Nobody had shoveled the sidewalk—footprints in the snow had partially melted and refrozen. No one had put out ice-melt. I slipped several times between my car and the front door and felt lucky to have stayed upright. I wondered how an elderly person would be able to navigate that route.

Inside the building, conditions weren't any better. The tables in the empty dining room were piled with dirty breakfast dishes. I looked at my watch. The posted schedule said they'd start serving lunch in less than an hour. I didn't see anyone in the office, but finally I tracked down the administrator, helping with a smelly clean-up in a hallway. She looked disheveled and unhappy.

"I'm sorry," she said. "We're short-handed today." I followed her to the office, and together we sorted through the records, finally pinpointing the source of the error.

Afterwards, I punched the code into the Alzheimer's unit door and entered the relative calm of that space. I saw Mom dozing in her room, so I peeked into the recreation room, where an aide sat, filling out paperwork. She looked exhausted.

"Are you okay?" I asked.

"Not really," she replied. "During this management turnover we've lost several good employees, and the rest of us are barely keeping up." She flashed me a wan smile. "But your mother had a really good day yesterday, and she's gained back two of the five pounds she lost."

**Saturday, December 31, 2016:** Since my employer closes operations between Christmas and New Year's, I've had some time to sift through most of my parents' files—the ones that I'd put aside because they weren't needed for their health care or legal proceedings. Much of it can be tossed, but I've found some of it quite fascinating, particularly my mother's family history research. When I visited her today, I did some 'name dropping' to see if any rang a bell with her. Most did not, but she seemed content to listen to me retelling the stories.

As I prepared to leave, a raised voice in the hallway caught my attention. I opened Mom's door a crack and peered out. A young man, perhaps in his late teens or early twenties, spoke harshly to an aide, who had her back against the wall.

"I won't let you treat my grandmother like this," he said. "She likes to exercise every day, play cards with her friends, read magazines, and cook great meals. Now she just sits; she acts like she doesn't even know who I am—I'm her favorite grandson. What have you done to her? Do you have her all drugged up?"

The aide's eyes widened as he took a step closer to her.

"Answer me!" he shouted.

Looking over my shoulder, I saw my mother asleep, so I stepped out into the hall and pulled the door shut. The aide saw me, eyes pleading for help. I looked up and down the corridor, but didn't see anyone.

"Excuse me," I said to the aide. "My mother is having some trouble. Can you please help us?"

She nodded and hurried after me into Mom's room. I closed the door.

My mother didn't stir, and the aide looked at me, her puzzled expression turning into one of gratitude.

"I know his grandmother," I said. "You are doing a good job. He doesn't understand what's happening to her."

**Saturday, January 7, 2017:** It's barely been above zero degrees for the past few days. But the roads are fine, so I paid Mom a visit.

When I arrived at the nursing home, I saw law enforcement, ambulances, and fire department vehicles idling in front of the main entrance. Concerned, I hurried inside. The receptionist told me that last night the pipes burst on the west side of the building, flooding patients' rooms with up to six inches of icy water. The police and fire officials were just finishing evacuating the residents from all the damaged rooms.

Seeing a look of alarm on my face, she reassured me that the Alzheimer's unit, on the building's east side, hadn't been affected. "We'd have called you if we needed to move your mother. It did get chilly inside the building for a while, but we bundled everyone up in blankets. Now the furnace is working again."

I proceeded to the locked unit and found my mother in the activity room, snoozing. She and several other residents wore sweaters and blankets around their shoulders, but none of them looked uncomfortable.

I sighed. This is just one more hurdle the staff has to deal with during the ownership transition. Although the change of ownership is technically complete, employees tell me they are still short-handed, and now this incident has relocated two-thirds of their residents, which may have catastrophic results on their revenue stream.

**Tuesday, February 28, 2017:** Despite the increase in my mother's income from Dad's pension and higher Social Security benefit, we are running out of money. The Veterans' Service Office has been assisting me since last May, trying to get my mother the benefits stemming from Dad's World War II service. The officer helping me passed away last week, unfortunately, so I'm not sure how that will affect this effort.

**Tuesday, March 14, 2017:** My mother turned eighty-eight years old today. I celebrated by attending a family conference and taking her to a series of medical appointments. Her cognition has deteriorated to the point where she no longer recognizes me at all. She remains physically functional. Since Mom likely won't know the difference, my husband and I are planning an end-of-the-month getaway to Florida.

**Sunday, April 9, 2017:** Barry and I are back from another trip to the southeast. We are trying to figure out what to do with his mother's house. We could keep it and retire there, but even though the weather is nice, we don't like the crowds. No matter, we aren't going anywhere as long as we have obligations in Nebraska.

# 36 CLARITY

**Monday, May 29, 2017:** Memorial Day. I went to see my mother. I detected no change in her mental or physical status. I think that, lately, I go to the nursing home more out of a sense of obligation than from any hope that she finds my visits meaningful. Today, she mostly slept while I was there, despite my efforts to wake her.

At least conditions at the facility finally seem improved after the rocky change of ownership. The center is once again fully staffed, repairs to the water-damaged rooms are complete, and the displaced residents have returned.

**Sunday, June 4, 2017:** This afternoon I made what I thought would be a quick run to O'Neill to visit Mom. To my surprise, she was wide awake when I entered her room, seated in the chair by the window. She looked at me with clear eyes and smiled.

"Hello, Sandy," she said distinctly.

Floored and delighted that she remembered me, I sat on the edge of her bed. We had a wonderful chat that must have lasted twenty minutes, until her fogginess returned.

Before leaving, I located an aide and told her that my mother had recognized me. "Has she been alert all day?"

The aide shook her head and said with an odd note of sadness in her voice, "No she hasn't. I'm so happy she knew you and that you had such a good visit."

I look forward to another visit next weekend.

**Thursday, June 8, 2017:** I spent today certifying forest thinning projects in the woods in the far western reaches of my work territory—close to three hours from my office. There is no cell service there, few people, and a lot of cattle. Perched in the shade of a ponderosa pine on the canyon rim, I ate lunch as I enjoyed the beautiful day and the breathtaking view of the river below. My mind kept wandering to my mother's mental clarity last weekend. Those thoughts remained with me as I resumed my tasks. When the sun sank toward the horizon, I reluctantly headed back toward civilization.

As I pulled into the parking space behind my office, I noticed a piece of white paper tacked to the back door. Thinking that odd, I pulled the note down and unfolded it. It said, "Sandy, call the nursing home in O'Neill. IMPORTANT!"

I unlocked the door and went inside, noticing a similar note taped to the glass on the front door. The answering machine showed several messages. Most were from the Four Seasons Nursing Home, asking me to phone them immediately. The last one, from Barry, also urged me to get hold of them.

With a gloomy premonition, I dialed their number. The social worker said, "Please sit down before we talk."

"Your mother has passed away. Her heart stopped while she sat in the dining room today. She died immediately, so even if we'd been able to reach you, there is no way you could have arrived in time. Please come right away."

I drove the forty-five minutes to O'Neill in a stupor. When I arrived at the nursing home, the social worker took me to Mom, lying peacefully on her bed, covered to the chin with a colorful afghan she had crocheted many years ago. I sat silently with her until the undertaker came and wheeled her away, leaving the afghan with me.

I remained motionless for a while and then mechanically began collecting her belongings. I could only find a few empty boxes, but I filled them, promising the staff I'd return for the rest tomorrow.

**Friday, June 9, 2017:** Barry helped me pack up the remainder of Mom's possessions and take them home. "This is your parents' final move," he said.

I nodded as I tried to count them. "I'm not entirely certain, but I think this is move number eleven. It's sure been quite a ride."

**Monday, June 12, 2017:** By now, Barry and I know exactly what to do when a parent dies, and we've been busy doing it. But the actual completion of these post-death tasks doesn't get any easier. Notifications, obituary, bill-paying, memorial service arrangements—it all just runs together in my head.

**Sunday, June 18, 2017:** This is my second Father's Day without Dad. Mom is with him now. I got a sympathy note from a logger who's worked on some of my forestry projects. His grandmother is in the same

Alzheimer's unit that housed my mother. I told him I'd given his grandma one of Mom's pretty shirts that his grandmother had often admired. I gave many of her other clothes to the nursing home after I learned that some residents don't have families to check on them.

**Monday, June 19, 2017:** A couple dozen people attended Mom's memorial service this morning. This time, I said 'yes' when Father Randy asked if I'd like to write a tribute, which I shared with the congregation. In part, this is what I said:

*My mother was a classy lady. Attractive and smart, she dressed well and always looked great. She had an engaging smile and a contagious laugh. When I was little, she could make me laugh until I cried. Sometimes we'd get the giggles, and Dad would roll his eyes and leave the room.*

*Mom was generous with both time and money. Her church was the center of her life. She volunteered without hesitation. For decades she taught Sunday school, led Bible studies, served on the church board, edited newsletters, and represented the parish at conventions. She worked tirelessly at a local museum, guided visitor tours, and taught safe driving classes for senior citizens. She epitomized the Energizer bunny.*

*Her generosity extended to me, too. Even during tough economic times, I never lacked for the basics. I remember her helping me with homework, despite her exhaustion after a tough day at work. When I was in college, I brought my dirty laundry home on long weekends and she insisted on washing it. She always sent me back with food, clean clothes, and extra spending money.*

*Mom loved entertaining and she enjoyed hosting fancy dinners. She'd mail hand-made invitations and spend hours poring over cookbooks to find just the right dish to serve. She made elaborate hors d'oeuvres and served drinks with little umbrellas in them. She made party favors and hand-lettered name cards for each place at the table. Every gathering had a theme, whether a Hawaiian luau or a red, white, and blue Fourth of July barbecue.*

*When my parents first moved to Bassett, I asked Mom why she didn't go to the senior center. "I'm not old enough," she told me (she was in her seventies at the time).*

*In her later years, Mom often said, "Getting old isn't for sissies." Cataract surgery helped failing vision for a while, but it became increasingly harder for her to do things such as thread a needle. Arthritis set in, and her joints became painful. For a long time she didn't let those things slow her down.*

*It's hard to watch someone you love decline and fade away. But her pain is gone now. A friend said, "She sure loved you. Not many moms would follow their kids all around the country." That's right. She loved me and I will be forever thankful for that.*

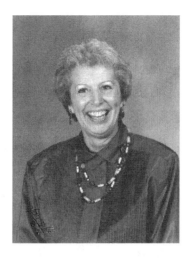

**Saturday, June 24, 2017:** I feel numb and empty—almost guilty, but not quite sure why. Although I'm still wrapping up my mother's affairs, I know that this process will end soon, leaving only memories, photos, and some keepsakes in its wake.

In the late 1800s, the German philosopher Friedrich Nietzsche coined what has since become an overused adage. Paraphrased, it says "That which doesn't kill us makes us stronger." Trite or not, I think this is an accurate statement of humankind's resilience in the face of adversity.

I believe my experiences over the past three years have indeed strengthened me and perhaps made me a bit wiser. I no longer harbor the resentment and bitterness I once did over the challenges I faced in just being my mother's daughter. I think that's why the eulogy I wrote for Mom was more than just 'making nice' because end-of-life tributes are supposed to be glowing. It's comforting to remember that she really did love me.

**Friday, August 25, 2017:** The battery on our landline telephone died, so I dug around in a box containing my parents' electronic devices and fished out one of their old handsets. I plugged it in and discovered it still works. I pushed the button to record a new greeting and heard my dad's voice, telling the caller that no one is here, so please leave a message. I didn't record a new message. It's nice to know that when I'm missing my father, I just have to push a button to hear his voice.

**Wednesday, September 6, 2017:** Saturday morning I'll be leaving to spend two weeks in the southwest. I'm taking my parents' ashes to the columbarium at the church they loved so much in Prescott, Arizona. After the commitment service, I'll travel to San Diego to see some cousins. While in California, I had hoped to visit Uncle George, my mom's brother, but he died last weekend. I imagine that losing both of her siblings this year has been hard on Aunt Virginia, their sister.

Someone recently asked me if my life has returned to normal. Absolutely not. I really haven't bounced back too well at all. I am just trying to keep on keeping on.

I understand that these things can take time—processing grief, recovering from the exhaustion of all the moves, doctors' and nursing home visits, and paperwork handled on my parents' behalf. The experience of witnessing their demises is something I'll not soon forget.

I have decided to turn this journal into a book. I will consider the time well spent, if my sharing of these experiences can help even one other person deal with the trauma that dementia can inflict on a family. Although I did, indeed, act as *My Mother's Keeper* for a time, my mother—in her own way—became my keeper as well.

# EPILOGUE
September 11, 2017—St. Luke's Episcopal Church, Prescott, Arizona

A handful of my parents' Arizona friends attended today's commitment service. The sun felt warm as we gathered in the church's memorial garden under a bright blue sky. One woman said, "We loved your folks, and we'll always remember how they brightened our lives. My children and I have talked, laughed, and quietly smiled so many times over the last thirty years because of them. God be with you, Lucy and George. We love you.".

Deacon Kimball prepared to place the two vessels containing my parents' ashes into the niche. She looked at me and asked, "Who should go in the front, your mom or your dad?"

"Mom," I replied without hesitation.

We all laughed, happy to know that my parents are finally home.

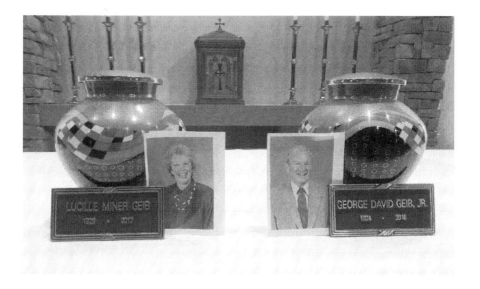

# ACKNOWLEDGMENTS

This, my first book, would not have been possible without many helping hands. These people fall into two groups: those who enabled me to survive the journey itself, and those who aided me in learning the ropes of becoming a published author.

My husband, Barry Benson, is the rock star of the first category. This book is dedicated to him. Other family members surrounded us with their support and love. My mother-in-law, Terry Benson, and my uncle, George Miner, provided us with much emotional sustenance. I regret they passed away before I published this story. Barry's uncles, George and Kenny Twist, were there for us throughout the ordeal.

Others, too, helped us endure. Father Randy Goeke offered spiritual guidance and the steadfast support of true friendship. Our friend and neighbor, Becky D., came through for us time and time again, helping with tasks both large and small, always with a smile and words of comfort. My classmate, Jill S.—who was going through her own parental situation at the same time—provided insight and an invaluable opportunity to compare notes and brainstorm coping strategies. Garrett Weidner, Warren Arganbright, and Mike O'Kief became the bridge that eventually got our family to the other side of the chasm. Many more friends—not named here for fear I'd miss some—provided ongoing moral support.

My employer and supervisors not only offered empathy, they made emergency family leave available to me, which allowed me to keep my job. And, of course, the dedicated staff at the nursing homes provided the tender yet professional care our elders needed until the end.

The second group includes those who encouraged me to get started on the book and to keep after it, even when reliving the memories made me want to quit. It also includes those who helped me put together and publish the book. The members of my local writers' group, the Ridgeline Literary Alliance, helped me look more critically at my writing style and techniques. I give a special shout out to Loren Leith, who taught me volumes about effective presentation, avoiding repetition, and eliminating clutter. Alex Peers helped with the pictures. Of course, thank you to Bob Grove, the best comma cop I've ever met. And thanks certainly go out to my beta readers, Lyn, Becky, John, Laurie, and Pam.

Thank goodness for my artist friends! Jill Spriggs created the cover art and Joan Swim made the map. Rachel Bostwick put the cover together. A special note of appreciation goes out to my editor, Debbie Manber Kupfer. She not only did a marvelous job editing, she also patiently taught me the basics of how to navigate the publishing world.

# FURTHER READING

As I muddled my way through our family's journey, I eventually stumbled upon a few resources that would have been more useful had I learned of them earlier. Initially, I thought I'd put a huge reference list at the end of this book. Since there's no point in reinventing the wheel, however, I've decided instead to build upon some excellent resources that already exist.

*The 36-Hour Day*, by Nancy L. Mace, M.A. and Peter V. Rabins, M.D., M.P.H. is probably the best-known comprehensive guide and is considered by many to be the gold standard dementia care handbook. First published in 1989, it is now in its sixth edition. It provides up-to-date information on dementias and their associated challenges for families and caregivers, as well as a synopsis of ongoing research. It includes an extensive resource listing. It is primarily a 'how-to' guide for families caring for a patient at home. I found the descriptions of dementia-induced behaviors particularly enlightening.

I highly recommend Jane Gross's book and the resource section at the end of it: *A Bittersweet Season: Caring for our Aging Parents and Ourselves*, Vintage 2012. This book combines the author's personal story with good descriptions of the facilities and people she encountered.

The book that might have been the most useful of all, had it been published in time, is *Creating Moments of Joy Along the Alzheimer's Journey: A Guide for Families and Caregivers*, by Jolene Brackey, 2017. The author's focus on the attitudes and understandings of caregivers is priceless. If I'd had such knowledge during my own journey, our family's life would have been much improved.

Many websites offer information and help for those caring for dementia patients. Try doing an internet search on text in the bullet points below. An internet search on a specific topic of inquiry will generally yield a large number of links. Here are a few samples:

- The Alzheimer's Reading Room: A Great Resource for Caregivers
- Better Health While Aging: Practical information for aging health and family caregivers
- HelpGuide Tips for Alzheimer's and Dementia Caregivers
- Home Care Assistance: Caring for a Parent with Dementia at Home

# ABOUT THE AUTHOR

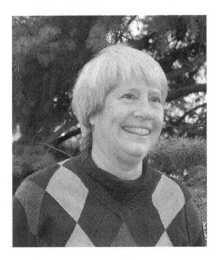

S. G. (Sandy) Benson writes from her home in the mountains of western North Carolina, where she lives with her husband, Barry, and two bossy dachshunds. A forester by training, she worked in the woods most of her life. Along the way, she published a real estate magazine and wrote many outdoors articles for newspapers and magazines. This is her first book. Eldercare was not even on her radar when the events described in this story began to unfold—it became an extraordinary learning experience. She says if this book helps even one person navigate the muddy waters of dementia, she'll consider it a success.

# TESTIMONIALS

"This book is incredible and the value the story can add for others going through a similar life event is unmeasurable. Towards the end the author says, "…if I can only help one other person…" MISSION ACCOM-PLISHED! I found this book exceptionally helpful in my recent journey with my mom and beyond. Understanding the journey we were on makes it sting a little less. It's an incredible story and a heartbreaking journey that needs to be shared with the world." —**John E., Lincoln, Nebraska**

"I couldn't put it down! It's a wonderful tribute to the family. I feel as if I've met them before, and I liked them all very much. The story provided the push to start on my own obituary which I've been meaning to do for a while now. And, yes, all those expenses—while I've given passing thought to them now and again—I may have to take a new look at our wills again to see if we can afford to die. The author is a most loving daughter." —**Laurie W., Hayesville, North Carolina**

"I'm a great fan of stories about polar explorations during the 19th and early 20th centuries. Often even the most well-prepared expeditions were ultimately doomed by the vagaries of weather, equipment reliability, and human personality. Men endured months (even years) of unrelenting cold and wet, limited sunlight, claustrophobic quarters, excruciatingly boring routines and too often succumbed to lead poisoning, snow blindness, frostbite resulting in loss of digits, starvation (sometimes cannibalism), and all kinds of mental aberrations. Yet, some did make it through. How much I have been awed by them!

Well, they have nothing on this journey. As I read the story I wondered, "HOW did she get through this?" I marvel at the physical, mental, spiritual, and moral strength manifested throughout those three years of hell. And with no one to blame for it! For me, the most poignant sentence in the whole story is "I feel like a monster." It almost made me cry. The author asked, "What can I do?" Well, no matter what she thought she did, she heroically gave what she could and well-served the four people closest to her. I can't imagine myself doing the same. The story really wore me out emotionally." —**Pam S., Crookston, Nebraska**

Made in the USA
Columbia, SC
27 November 2021

49755124R00065